Praise for *Beauty Secrets*

"This fabulous, practical book offers a healthier view of beauty for the Christian woman. The recommendations and recipes are easy to follow, as well as medically and spiritually sound. Garrett strips away the layers of dead myths and expectations, providing wonderful beauty alternatives and giving you permission to cherish yourself the way God intended.

—CARRIE L. CARTER, M.D., author of *A Woman's Guide to Good Health*

"If you've never thought of the Bible as a beauty manual, think again. Ginger Garrett has lovingly and wittily gleaned the Bible's wisdom, providing easy-to-follow advice on foods, oils, and perfumes that will let you create a healthy, glowing body naturally and inexpensively. Most importantly, *Beauty Secrets of the Bible* teaches us to rejoice in the body we have."

—INDIA EDGHILL, author of *Wisdom's Daughter: A Novel of Solomon and Sheba*

"Ginger Garrett's book is filled with powerful, precise, and ancient beauty ritual secrets fit not just for celebrities, but for everyone to experience. A must read!"

—CHRISTOPHER WATT, celebrity skin care expert, founder of Christopher Watt Esthetics, and CEO of CWE Skincare, Inc.

"In a culture that seduces women with $35 one-ounce vials of 'miracle' lotions and potions, who would guess that the answer to so many beauty concerns can be found in one's own pantry? And for a fraction of the cost! Ginger Garrett not only frees up our credit cards by letting us in on ancient beauty secrets that are sure to hit the cosmetic industry in its collective pocketbook, but backs them up with research. And did I mention the daily devotions? Beauty outside *and* in!"

—TAMARA LEIGH, author of *Perfecting Kate* and *Splitting Harriet*

"Garrett's beauty regime is the simplest in the world. But watch out: it's life-changing! This book will challenge you to view yourself the way your Creator does."

—SIRI L. MITCHELL, author of *Kissing Adrien*

"Ginger Garrett's book gave me exactly what I needed—a devotional that reflects what God determines as real beauty and a guide to the beauty secrets of the Bible. I checked the labels on the skin care and makeup items I currently use, and then rushed out to make my own or replace them with natural products. What a delightful eye opener."

—DIANN MILLS, author of *The Texas Legacy* series and *When the Nile Runs Red*

"As a former licensed cosmetologist, I found Ginger Garrett's *Beauty Secrets of the Bible* to be intriguing, practical, and most of all, wise."

—LYN COTE, author of *Blessed Assurance*

"Ginger Garrett has captured true, authentic beauty in this wonderful book. The focus on organic products and homemade remedies is extremely beneficial to the health, beauty, and well-being of all women.

—KIMBERLY SAYER, CEO and founder of Kimberly Sayer of London (producer of organic skin care products)

Beauty Secrets of the Bible

The Ancient Arts of Beauty & Fragrance

GINGER GARRETT

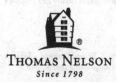

THOMAS NELSON
Since 1798

NASHVILLE DALLAS MEXICO CITY RIO DE JANEIRO BEIJING

Published in Nashville, Tennessee, by Thomas Nelson. Thomas Nelson is a registered trademark of Thomas Nelson, Inc.

Thomas Nelson, Inc., titles may be purchased in bulk for educational, business, fund-raising, or sales promotional use. For information, please e-mail SpecialMarkets@ThomasNelson.com.

All Scripture quotations, unless otherwise indicated, are taken from the New King James Version®. Copyright © 1982 by Thomas Nelson, Inc. Used by permission. All rights reserved.

Scripture quotations marked NCV are taken from The New Century Version®. Copyright © 2005 by Thomas Nelson, Inc. Used by permission. All rights reserved.

Scriptures marked NIV are taken from THE HOLY BIBLE, NEW INTERNATIONAL VERSION®. NIV®. Copyright ©1973, 1978, 1984 by International Bible Society. Used by permission of Zondervan. All rights reserved.

Scriptures marked KJV are taken from The King James Version of the Bible.

Scriptures marked MSG are taken from *The Message* by Eugene H. Peterson, copyright © 1993, 1994, 1995, 1996, 2000, 2001, 2002. Used by permission of NavPress Publishing Group. All rights reserved.

Every effort has been made to make this book as accurate as possible. The purpose of this book is to educate. It is a review of scientific evidence that is presented for information purposes. No individual should use the information in this book for self-diagnosis, treatment, or justification in accepting or declining any medical therapy for any health problems or diseases.

No individual is discouraged from seeking professional medical advice and treatment, and this book is not supplying medical advice. Any application of the information herein is at the reader's own discretion and risk. Therefore, any individual with a specific health problem or who is taking medications must first seek advice from his or her personal physician or health-care provider before starting a nutrition program. The author and Thomas Nelson Publishers, Inc., shall have neither liability nor responsibility to any person or entity with respect to loss, damage, or injury caused or alleged to be caused directly or indirectly by the information contained in this book. We assume no responsibility for errors, inaccuracies, omissions, or any inconsistency herein.

In view of the complex, individual nature of health and fitness problems, this book, and the ideas, programs, procedures, and suggestions are not intended to replace the advice of trained medical professionals. All matters regarding one's health require medical supervision. A physician should be consulted prior to adopting any program or programs described in this book. The author and publisher disclaim any liability arising directly or indirectly from the use of this book.

The author and publisher have presented the websites listed in the Resource Guide for reference only, and are not responsible for the content of these external websites. The author and publisher do not operate or control in any respect any information, products, or services on such sites. References to any such sites shall not be taken as an endorsement by the author or publisher of opinions expressed or services provided at those sites.

Author is represented by the literary agency of Alive Communications, Inc., 7680 Goddard Street, Suite 200, Colorado Springs, Colorado 80920.

Library of Congress Cataloging-in-Publication Data

Garrett, Ginger, 1968–
    Beauty secrets of the Bible : the ancient arts of beauty and fragrance
/ Ginger Garrett.
        p. cm.
    Includes bibliographical references.
    ISBN: 978-0-7852-2178-4
    1. Beauty, Personal—Biblical teaching. 2. Beauty, Personal—Religious aspects—Christianity.
3. Women—Health and hygiene. 4. Herbal cosmetics. I. Title.
RA778.G344 2007
646.7'042—dc22   2007004617

Printed in the United States of America
08 09 10 11 12 QW 7 6 5 4 3

For Andi

Contents

Introduction

I stumbled upon the lost beauty secrets of the Bible in my
career as a novelist. As I researched my first novel, *Chosen: The
Lost Diaries of Queen Esther*, which was based on the legendary
queen who devoted a year of her life to beauty, I was curious
about what sort of treatments would have been available to
women nearly 3,000 years ago.

To my amazement, I discovered that the beauty treatments of
our ancient sisters rivaled our own. In some ways, these treatments were even superior, free of harmful synthetic chemicals
and preservatives. And almost every product used long, long ago
is being "rediscovered" today by the beauty industry. This book
will unlock the secrets of those ancient women, the women of the
biblical lands who still whisper to us from the past.

Every woman deserves to look and feel her best, just as God
created her. This book is not only about rediscovering ancient
secrets from our sisters; it's also about rediscovering our own
beauty. Modern beauty has become heavily commercialized—it's
a one-hundred-billion-dollars-a-year industry. (Estimates put the

beauty/personal care industry at $35 billion per year in the United States, and the weight loss industry at approximately $65 billion.) These industries fuel multimillion dollar ad campaigns that encourage us to embrace a commercial standard of beauty, not our own authentic artistry. When we lose touch with our true selves, we lose touch with the spiritual nature of God's design, and His unique artistry expressed through us.

My prayer is that this book will help set you free: free from expensive, misleading products, free from oppressive cultural messages, and free to discover who you were meant to be. I'll teach you how to create the most luxurious, exclusive skin care and beauty regimen imaginable—one that will give you real results. Best of all, you can save over $1,500 this year by making these simple, healthy choices.

We are spirits living in a body, and how we care for that body is a reflection of the spirit-life within. Come with me on a journey of exploring the unique relationship between worshiping our Creator and caring for ourselves. Come with me as we shake off the deception and lies of a commercial industry out of control.

Come with me into the forgotten world of the *Beauty Secrets of the Bible.*

❧ 1 ❧

Twenty-Eight Days
of Cleansing

The first step of any beauty regimen is cleansing. Interestingly, it is also the first step in approaching God. Jewish priests at the temple had to begin with ceremonial washing before they could attend to their calling, just as Christ's sacrifice washes His believers so that they can be presented to God as without stain or spot.

Beauty, both physical and spiritual, is a profound and often troubling concept. To discover what it really means, we need to begin by washing away what is not of our authentic selves—the pollution and dead layers of anxiety, fear, and loneliness. We must bring to the surface of our souls what we truly feel and think about beauty, so that our minds and hearts can at last be at peace with our spirits and discover a more meaningful path than the one presented to us by society.

We'll begin the journey to the heart of true beauty with a cleansing. For twenty-eight days, you are encouraged to read one meditation a day and to reflect on it. You may read the meditations one by one before going on to begin the book, or read the meditations in between readings from the book.

And let the beauty of the LORD our God be upon us. . . .
—PSALM 90:17

$\mathcal{T}$he first beauty secret of the Bible is that it's not only okay to believe yourself to be beautiful, but that belief—that you are beautiful—is actually part of your spiritual life. Beauty is an expression of spiritual creativity. Beauty originates with God. It is a definition of God and a focal point of our praise. And while many women worship God and have an intimate, thriving relationship with Him, only 2 percent of women consider themselves beautiful.[1] Where is the disconnect in our culture? Where is the disconnect within you and me?

The world believes beauty is an external varnish and a temporary condition. But in reality, beauty is woven into our being; it is not created every morning in front of the mirror. Beauty is our spiritual birthright.

Beauty is not about what we're presenting—a finished product to be judged—but what we're expressing. Beauty communicates the state of our spirit. It is the language of the spiritual world. The standards of earthly beauty change through time and culture, but the pursuit of beauty is universal and timeless.

Again, I'm not simply talking about "billboard beauty." That's a manipulated image of beauty, an oppressive, silent indictment of the majority of women who don't measure up. What we'll be talking about in this book is the creative, healthy, outward manifestation of a beautiful life within, the spirit of God who dwells in us. We are women who are deeply loved and beautiful by His touch.

Ask: God, what does "beauty" mean to me, and why do I desire it?

Believe: I am beautiful by His touch.

Day Two: ACKNOWLEDGING THE WOUND

. . . He made us accepted in the Beloved.

—EPHESIANS 1:6

$\mathcal{A}$t the heart of every woman afraid to call herself beautiful is a woman who has been wounded. Avoiding beauty, or refusing to pursue it, is self-protection. In our hearts we believe we'll never be good enough, that we'll never be accepted. Our efforts are half-hearted. For years, my only goal was to avoid humiliation. I didn't want to feel the pain of my childhood, when I was called a monster and bullied into believing I was, and forever would be, ugly. I was not accepted. How could I ever call myself beautiful?

In those childhood years, I read a fairy tale about a mermaid girl who longed to be beautiful. Her mother clipped shells on her tail, and as the girl cried out, her mother reminded her that beauty must hurt. Today I see that is a true statement for so many of us. Beauty does hurt, but for a different reason: it hurts to open ourselves again to disappointment and rejection. Acknowledging our desire for beauty can reopen wounds we've fought to close. We wanted silence to heal us and avoidance to make us forget. But the little girl who longed to be beautiful, to be accepted, is still inside. What are we to do with her?

In Luke 18:16, Jesus said, "Let the little children come to Me, and do not forbid them; for of such is the kingdom of God." Are you willing to bring the little girl inside you to Jesus? He will accept her just as she is. He will protect her and give her the courage to believe again. To allow her to believe again in love and beauty, and in a God who will always call her Beautiful.

> *Ask:* God, heal my wounds.
>
> *Believe:* In Jesus I'm healed and unconditionally accepted.

"Abide in Me, and I in you.
As the branch cannot bear fruit of itself, unless it abides in the vine,
neither can you, unless you abide in Me. . . .
As the Father loved Me, I also have loved you; abide in My love."
—JOHN 15:4, 9

Dr. Hema Sundaram, dermatologist, cosmetic surgeon, and author of *Face Value: The Truth About Beauty—and a Guilt-Free Guide to Finding It*, told me that, many times, women fear "divine retribution" if they seek to alter or improve their appearance. "They may feel guilt or shame, and project this onto God," she said.

We have strong emotional reactions to the subject of beauty and the possibility of altering our appearance in any way. Some of us insist that anything is acceptable as long as it makes us feel good. Others insist God intended for us to be all-natural—no makeup, no surgery, no elaborate clothes or jewelry. This fierce emotional reaction is evidence that our beauty is close to the marrow of our souls.

Women are afraid of losing love: we're afraid God will reject us if we overvalue our appearance, and we're afraid others will reject us if we don't value it enough. But Jesus reassures us that our lives are rooted in His love for us. It is this love that is the source of all good things in our lives, including true beauty. As we root deeply into the Source of life and love, beauty will be a natural by-product of our efforts. Worry lines will soften. We'll stop turning to the refrigerator for comfort so often. Our faces will have a soft glow of contentment and peace that is more alluring than any cosmetic.

Any desire of our hearts—even the desire to be physically beautiful—is an invitation for God to reveal Himself to us. By bringing this desire to God, we are moving beauty out of the shadows and into the light. We can trust that God will teach us in this journey to root deeply down into His love.

Ask: God, reveal to me the true source of beauty.

Believe: God is using my desire for beauty to teach me about His constant, unconditional love and affection.

> *Trust in the LORD with all your heart,*
> *And lean not on your own understanding;*
> *In all your ways acknowledge Him,*
> *And He shall direct your paths.*
>
> —PROVERBS 3:5–6

Rabbi Efraim Davidson of the DoJewish Campaign of Atlanta spoke with me about the legacy of beauty and faith. "When the Jews were enslaved in Egypt," he explained, "the men were humiliated all day long, degraded. The women took special care to make themselves look beautiful, so that when their husbands came home, they felt respected. It made them feel human again." Beauty was not about how the women judged themselves, but the effect it had on those around them. It reached the men's souls where words could not.

"Later," Rabbi Davidson tells us, "when the Jews were freed from their slavery, the women gave their mirrors to be used in constructing the tabernacle." Beauty had been a sacred service that honored God. Beauty was indeed a part of their worship, a way to honor God in their physical lives, and a winsome reminder that our earthly lives can be given in sacred service in many ways. You can reach for God, even in this distinctly feminine preoccupation, and confidently expect Him to take hold of you and lead you into a safe and honored place.

As we talk about beauty in this book, let go of all your preconceived notions about what beauty is and is not. "Lean not on your own understanding," but ask God to reveal Himself in everything.

Ask: God, help me to let go of my own answers and seek Yours instead.

Believe: God will use the questions of beauty to bless my life richly, in ways I cannot imagine yet.

"The lamp of the body is the eye. If therefore your eye is good,
your whole body will be full of light.
But if your eye is bad, your whole body will be full of darkness. . . ."
—MATTHEW 6:22–23

Our eyes bring either light or darkness into the body. Jesus spoke these words to introduce the idea that we reside either in the darkness or in the light, depending on our vision. A woman with a vision of God lives in the light. A woman focused only on herself only lives in darkness. Jesus used eyes as a metaphor for our spiritual lives: eyes are an entry point that affects the whole being.

Jesus also taught, in Matthew 5:29, that what our eyes focus on can affect our spirit and lead us into sin. Our physical eyes can be described as spiritually neutral, but Jesus warns us they are incredibly powerful, for they are capable of affecting our inner life. Haven't you experienced seeing an image that permeates your thinking and continually pops into your mind, unwanted? Do you find yourself wishing you had never seen it, but that now it is a part of you? Jesus uses our eyes to teach us that our souls and spirits are captive to our physical lives and habits.

We are spirits, and souls, living within bodies. What affects one affects all three. Only death can separate the three. (The traditional interpretation of *spirit* versus *soul* is that *spirit* refers to our immortal beings and the *soul* to our earthly intellect and emotions.)

Beauty is a physical manifestation of the spirit and soul, and the spirit and soul are held captive by our physical choices. Therefore, the greatest of care should be given to how we care for ourselves, and why. We understand beauty as a metaphor for God and honor it as such, but we also acknowledge that the act of creating physical beauty can have a spiritual impact as well.

Ask: God, show me where I am making unwise choices in my life.

Believe: Others see the outward radiance of my inner life.

[The Beloved speaks:] "Like a lily among thorns,
So is my love among the daughters."
[The Bride replies:] "Like an apple tree among the trees of the woods,
So is my beloved among the sons.
I sat down in his shade with great delight, and his fruit was sweet to my taste. . . .
Set me as a seal upon your heart, as a seal upon your arm;
For love is as strong as death. . . ."
—SONG OF SOLOMON 2:2–3, 8:6

*B*eauty serves a practical purpose in a divine world: beauty attracts us.

In a crowded room, we gravitate toward what attracts us. In a crowded world, there is no neutrality; we move toward beauty. All of the natural world operates on this principle. Beautiful colors attract bees and birds to flowers. Humans instinctively turn toward the sunrise and sunset and inhale quietly as we mark another passage of time by the beauty of the skies. Beauty orients us in the world, pulls us in, and pushes us to search for what has been lost. We want to surround ourselves with it, lavish in it, and soothe our frazzled nerves by it.

But beauty only begins the foundational work of love. A single stone is not a building but a beginning. It can offer no shelter, no warmth, no rest. Likewise, beauty can only offer itself to be built upon. What we build on it—deep, lasting love—is a force as strong as death itself.

Beauty attracts us, but it is the love we build on it that makes us truly beautiful in another's eyes. Physical beauty is a lovely spark that catches the eye but disappears in a moment's breath. It is love that catches the spark and feeds it, fans it, until it glows and burns, creating a steady fire that lights a new generation.

Ask: God, show me how to build love in my life.

Believe: Love makes me incredibly beautiful, and God promises I am incredibly loved.

But we all, with unveiled face, beholding as in a mirror the glory of the LORD,
are being transformed into the same image from glory to glory,
just as by the Spirit of the LORD.

—2 CORINTHIANS 3:18

*B*eauty is entwined with love. Both herald the eternal. As we experience love, we are transformed, tasting the eternal. Think of a first true love, or the first moment you held your baby in your arms. The beauty of your loved one was overwhelming to you, immeasurable. The outside world meant nothing in that moment. Cynicism was dead.

It's no coincidence that at these moments in our lives, we turn to God. Engaged couples seek the blessing of a minister and brand-new parents reinvestigate forgotten faith. Love has made our beloved beautiful to us, and at that moment, we are open to believe in the eternal. Our hearts are opened to believe in God even if we've drifted away. Beauty calls us home.

Will you experience the beautiful today? Will you feel the sun on your arms and marvel at the theater of lights above you at night? Will you delight in the construction of a flower and know yourself to be a part of this same creation? Will you love someone from the depths of your heart and see God's beauty? Will you allow yourself to look in the mirror and see a woman made beautiful in love? Beauty and love are deeply entwined in this life and the next.

> *Ask:* God, break through the cynicism and fear guarding my heart and let me know love and see beauty.
>
> *Believe:* I am so deeply loved that I radiate beauty and attract others.

For now we see in a mirror, dimly, but then [in heaven] face to face.
Now I know in part, but then I shall know just as I also am known.

—I CORINTHIANS 13:12

$\mathcal{T}$oday we see with clouded vision and long for a time when our eyes will be opened and paradise entered into again.

Our efforts to be beautiful will always be somewhat frustrated on earth. We will never reach a moment when we feel the completion of beauty and know ourselves to be finally, forever, beautiful. The longing we feel for beauty will always be kindled, just as a longing for rest is always with us. Beauty whets our appetite for its final fulfillment.

When you are frustrated with your appearance, remember it is not because your body or beauty lacks something. It is because the world lacks something. The quest for perfection isn't a vain desire but a shadow of a greater desire, the first desire—the desire to be unashamed before God and man, to reflect completely the love of the Creator as He beholds us.

Ask: Help me to gracefully accept this desire that will never be fully satisfied on earth.

Believe: Someday God's perfect beauty will be made complete in me.

> *But the LORD said to Samuel,*
> *"Do not look at his appearance or at his physical stature, because I have refused him.*
> *For the LORD does not see as man sees;*
> *for man looks at the outward appearance, but the LORD looks at the heart."*
>
> —I SAMUEL 16:7

Of all the women noted in Scripture as physically beautiful, can you tell me what any one of them looked like?

I can't either. No physical quality is accurately described. Women are simply said to be lovely in form, or beautiful. The text is always purposely vague. God avoids telling us the particulars. Why would God tell us that women in Scripture were physically beautiful, but never tell us what they looked like?

Perhaps God is hinting that when we claim a woman is beautiful, we also hint that others are less so. We would be oppressed for all time if the beautiful women of the Bible were accurately described, because our tendency is to believe there is but one standard for physical beauty. As a culture, we instinctively move toward one ideal while we reject all others. We are wired for worship, and it spills over even into our consideration of appearance.

God acknowledges that some women are considered in their time as beautiful. God doesn't define their physical beauty. He leaves it a mystery. Yet we know God is a very specific builder: He gives exact measurements for His creations, including the temple, the ark of the covenant, and Noah's ark. For these, He lists specific materials and colors to be used, types of wood, fabric, jewels, shapes, designs, and fragrances. But not once does He define the ideal shape, size, color, or appearance of a beautiful woman. Let's take the same approach. Let's stop defining beauty in absolute, worldly terms. Let's leave it a mystery.

Ask: God, give me the willingness to surrender my ideas about beauty.

Believe: I will see the beauty in all women and celebrate that beauty.

For as she thinks in her heart, so is she.
—PROVERBS 23:7 (AUTHOR'S PARAPHRASE)

With repeated exposure to harmful, degrading messages about our appearance and weight, we become maimed and lessened in our souls. We see the finished product of advertising and feel frustration. We are real women, with real lives. Nobody's standing around to airbrush us or check for stray hairs. The older we get, the further we move from the "ideal," and we become further disenfranchised from beauty. We have spent our lives being told beauty was only just beyond our reach; now we are told it is lost to us forever.

When we allow someone else to set our expectations, we allow someone else to control our destiny. Expectations are powerful precursors to action. A wise man once told me that in life, "your expectations will be met." Expectations condition us to respond and receive. Expectations are deeply connected to our thoughts, and these thoughts shape our destiny.

If you believe beauty is within you, no matter how it is manifested on the outside, you will see yourself as beautiful. Others will respond this way as well. You create a self-fulfilling prophecy with every bit of inner dialogue. If you tell yourself you don't measure up, you won't. You'll fall short and cringe when people look closely at you. You'll shy away from your birthright. The world wants to set your expectations for you and to whisper to you degrading beliefs about yourself, because fearful women make millions of dollars for callous companies.

Can you find the courage to defy the world and change your expectations? Can you expect to be pleased when you see yourself in the mirror tomorrow morning? Can you expect to be loved and accepted?

> *Ask:* God, reset my expectations.
>
> *Believe:* I expect to see the beauty in myself.

> *"Now if God so clothes the grass of the field,*
> *which today is, and tomorrow is thrown into the oven,*
> *will He not much more clothe you, O you of little faith?"*
> —MATTHEW 6:30

Women are multitaskers. We tie the children's shoes, make the appointments, brew the coffee, pay the bills, cook a meal, clean the house, run our careers, keep our men happy, care for aging parents, and serve in the church. In our spare time, we nurture a relationship with God and find time to exercise and get our nails done. Whew! It's not enough that we expect ourselves to be able to run the world: we expect that we will look fabulous while doing it. We expect a lot from ourselves, don't we?

We expect a lot from physical beauty, too. We expect that physical beauty will bring us many things, but most importantly, we expect beauty to bring us love and acceptance. After all, these core desires are what we were designed for. We absolutely crave love and acceptance, and the root of these yearnings is in our spirits.

No one craves what they have never tasted. We crave love and acceptance because our spirits once knew complete acceptance and unconditional love through intimacy with God. We cannot manufacture a cure for this craving, because humanity is not the source. God is. Only God can satisfy the hunger.

Let go of your expectations of what physical beauty could bring you. God is the source of all good gifts. You may never have a supermodel's body or face. You may be confined to a wheelchair, or have scars that cannot be healed. Yet nothing can stop God from giving you what He wants to give you. If God lovingly attends to even the grass, which is of no value, how much more will He do for you?

Let God give you what you crave. No one multitasks like He can!

Ask: What is it that You want to give me, that I can't get from physical beauty?

Believe: I trust God to bring me all good gifts.

> *Your eyes will see the King in His beauty.* . . .
> —ISAIAH 33:17

> *He has no form or comeliness; And when we see Him,*
> *There is no beauty that we should desire Him.*
> *He is despised and rejected by men,*
> *A Man of sorrows and acquainted with grief.*
> —ISAIAH 53:2–3

*I*n Scripture, Christ is both referred to as beautiful and radiant and also as not beautiful, even disturbing, to look at. The apparent contradiction has spurred debate; does beauty lead us to God, or does suffering? Is God found best in pain or in ecstasy? Who has a better idea of the deeper spiritual truths: someone who contemplates beauty, or the one who contemplates the pains of the world?

The message of Christ is, perhaps, that both views lead us to God at different points in our journey. Christ is radiant and beautiful, but to suffer in our place, He had to absorb the painful sin we were soiled with. He is the same Christ in beauty as in disfigurement, and we can know Him in either pain or ecstasy.

The concepts of beauty and ugliness are not opposites, but different points on the continuum of eternity. God is total beauty, beauty that crucified our disfigurement. In His beauty we will see the ugliness of a world without Him, and in the ugliness of the world we find the beauty of God.

Ask: Teach me to see You in both beauty and pain.

Believe: Beauty surrounds me where I least expect to find it.

> *He causes the grass to grow for the cattle, And vegetation for the service of man,*
> *That he may bring forth food from the earth . . . [and] oil to make his face shine.*
> —PSALM 104:14–15

*I*n biblical days, grooming and maintaining a clean appearance reflected our joy with the Creator. Rubbing the face with oil, often called the "oil of gladness," was seen as a pleasurable gift from God that made the face glow with health. Using the oil of gladness was a sign that life was, indeed, good. Having a radiant face was also the direct result of intimacy with God. Moses, after spending time in the Lord's presence on Mount Sinai, was said to be so radiant that he had to cover his face. Everything associated with God is radiant:

> His commands are radiant (Ps. 19:8).
> His angels are radiant (Rev. 10:1–3).
> His robes are radiant (Mark 9:2–4).
> God is radiance, and everything emanating from God or in His
>   presence is touched by this same light: the land is radiant
>   with His glory (Ezek. 43:1–3).
> Those who look to Him are radiant (Ps. 34: 4–5).

Radiance is not dependent on the mechanics of outer construction: there is no mention of proportions between noses and eyes, hair colors and skin colors. In the Lord's presence, there is simply the beauty of radiance. How lovely to think of a spiritual world just beyond our own where racism and judgment no longer exist, replaced by a radiance that allows us only to see the light of God reflected on each other's faces.

Ask: Bless me with Your radiance.

Believe: When people see me, they will see the radiance of love and gladness.

> *"No servant can serve two masters;*
> *for either he will hate the one and love the other,*
> *or else he will be loyal to the one and despise the other."*
> —LUKE 16:13

*I*f you feel a little uneasy talking about beauty and spirituality, that's okay. There is an unnatural, uneasy relationship in our society between the two. In biblical days, it was easier to understand the symbolism of caring for the body in relationship to the state of your spirit. Before you could worship, you had to ceremonially wash yourself. Applying oil and perfume was a sign of blessing, an anointing that often meant much more than mere grooming. You were preparing to go into God's holy presence, the temple's sacred ground. To prepare the body was to prepare to meet God.

What do you think of today as you prepare your body in the mornings, even on the mornings you prepare for church? I think about wrinkles, cellulite, pore size, plump lips, and expertly lined eyes. I'm preparing for someone, but is it God? Truthfully, I want to greet the world and know that it approves of my appearance. I want to please God *and* the world. But this journey I've been on has pushed me to continually choose between the two desires. For as much as we talk about tolerance in our culture, there is no middle ground when it comes to our spiritual lives: we can't tolerate competing spiritual desires.

If we want to discover the beauty that God created in us, we have to be willing to abandon the world's definition of beauty. We have to believe, by faith, that we have something more: a beauty that cannot be fully seen by human eyes.

Ask: Show me how preparing myself to greet the world is really a preparation to meet You.

Believe: I prepare myself in the expectation of seeing God's love today.

> *Splendor and beauty mark his craft;*
> *His generosity never gives out.* . . . *His miracles are his memorial—*
> *This GOD of Grace, this GOD of Love.*
> —PSALM 111:3–4 MSG

*H*ow would you say the world defines *beauty?* I think the world defines it in one word, and I think this word also sums up why some women "let themselves go." The word is *seduction,* the power of luring a man into an illicit encounter. Of course, then, we feel uneasy talking about beauty when the culture's subtext is that beauty is only crafted for seduction. And if we've been blessed to find satisfying marriages with good men, we often feel that worldly ideas about illicit seduction have little place in marriage. We begin to think beauty isn't all that important to us.

But what if beauty was rooted in sacrificial love, not seduction? Would we consider someone else's feelings as we cared for our appearance? Great beauty, like great love, is demonstrated best in the sacrifices we make.

I collect vintage and costume jewelry, exotic but inexpensive pieces. I wore my newest prize one day, a stunning silver necklace. When a friend admired it, I felt an unwelcome tug in my spirit: I had the distinct impression God wanted me to take it off and give it to her. So I did, amid much internal wailing and gnashing of teeth. But when it was glittering in her palm instead of on my neck, I felt a burst of freedom, joy, and peace. I wanted that necklace to make me look good; without it, I felt more beautiful than I had in years.

You are a miracle of stunning design, too, formed in the dark quiet of an unseen womb, created to display the grace of God to a dying world. You are a memorial to the God of love. Your life is a sacrifice to offer Him, and your beauty is an invitation to others to know and be known.

Ask: Teach me that spirit is the root of life, and love is the root of beauty.

Believe: Physical beauty isn't about what I can get from the world. True beauty is about what I can give.

> *Your beauty, within and without, is absolute, dear lover, close companion.*
>
> —SONG OF SOLOMON 7:6 MSG

*H*ave you ever been deeply, unconditionally loved? Did you feel beautiful and secure? When we don't feel loved, we're insecure about our beauty. We're insecure about our place in the world.

The question, "do you think I'm beautiful?" is ultimately a question of "do you love me?" We cannot make peace with our appearance if we feel unloved. Without love, our eyes are clouded and what we see when we look in the mirror is not an adequate reflection of who we are, or even how we truly appear to others.

But we cannot depend on love, at least not the love most girls are encouraged to believe in—the romantic, never-failing passion of a knight and princess. In this world, knights fall off their horses quite regularly, and princesses are too busy doing their taxes to hang around windows and let down their hair. In the real world, husbands sometimes find new wives. Disease and disaster end the story too soon. Even the best earthly love is not a lifetime guarantee.

But God's love doesn't change. He loves us with a strength we cannot fathom, and one I cannot describe. His love covers the gaps. His heavenly love makes it possible to love on earth. In God, we are loved. We are beautiful. When we age and our bodies fill out even as our faces grow taut, He still sees the beauty in us. Where there are gaps in our love, He closes them. Where we lack or tremble, He fills and steadies.

> *Ask:* Help me to believe I am Your beloved, safe with You for all of eternity.
>
> *Believe:* I am safe and loved. This relationship with God will never end.

> *. . . as the bridegroom rejoices over the bride,*
> *So shall your God rejoice over you.*
>
> —ISAIAH 62:5

This is the heart of physical beauty in a spiritual world: that we adorn ourselves in expectation of seeing the One who gave His life for us. We'll see Him today in the faces of strangers or in the smile of a child, and someday we'll see Him, His hands outstretched, ready to welcome us home. Every day is a wedding day, as God rejoices over us as His bride, a woman He calls beautiful, a woman He calls His own.

Beauty is expectation. We don't bother with our appearance when we don't expect to see someone. How you groom yourself today reveals what you expect and what you hope for.

But what about those of us who feel unloved? Intellectually, we can understand that God calls us His beloved bride, a woman He has made beautiful. But some of us can't feel it and the truth doesn't penetrate our hearts. This hidden shame is rooted in fear that we don't measure up, despite God's affirmations.

Second Timothy 1:7 reminds us that "God has not given us a spirit of fear, but of power and of love and of a sound mind." This fear we carry is not from God, dear sister. We must reject it at every turn. We *are* the beloved bride, and we are not meant to sit out our own wedding feast. God wants us to experience His love as more than intellectual truth. Whatever is holding you back today, confess it. Name the fears that drive you away from His arms. Give up whatever keeps you searching elsewhere for affirmation and beauty. God has given you the power to believe and a sound mind to recognize and accept the truth. Through Christ, God has done more than proclaim His love for you: He's given you the power to fully receive it.

Ask: Help me fully accept Your embrace.

Believe: I am opening the door of my heart: I am welcoming Love into every dark corner.

Surely goodness and mercy shall follow me all the days of my life.
—PSALM 23:6

*H*ow do we behave when we've ordered an item and are waiting for it to be delivered?

Do we fly into a rage when we see the item advertised on TV? Do we resent our neighbor who already has one? Do we plead with God, or denounce Him, because He hasn't given it to us? Of course not— we simply wait for it to arrive. We expect. We aren't afraid to kindle our desire or acknowledge it, for we anticipate that at any moment the desire will be fulfilled.

What is it you are expecting today as you read this book? Contemplating physical and spiritual beauty can bring up the core fears and hopes in our hearts. We may find ourselves sneaking the time to read, afraid to acknowledge openly that we want to be beautiful. Or, we may find ourselves frantically turning pages, searching for the one passage that will illuminate our distress so we can be free at last.

We all have expectations, whether we're reading a book or choosing a laundry detergent. Today, watch how you behave as you read and think about beauty. Observe how you interact with other women and how you react when you see yourself in a mirror. How you act will tell you a lot about what you believe.

The truth is, no matter what you believe, God's goodness and mercy are following you, right here, right now. You don't have to ask for it, to order it, or to remind God to deliver it. It's a done deal, signed, sealed, and heading straight for you. You already have what you desperately want.

Ask: Help me believe Your beauty and love are indeed mine already.

Believe: Goodness and mercy surround me in everything I do.

---

*"The thief does not come except to steal, and to kill, and to destroy.
I have come that they may have life, and that they may have it more abundantly."*
—JOHN 10:10

*Your vibrant beauty has gotten inside us—you've been so good to us! We're walking on
air! All we are and have we owe to GOD, Holy God of Israel, our King!*
—PSALM 89:17–18 MSG

Who defines beauty?

In this world, beauty is defined as something apart from God, a force
for seducing, manipulating, and securing admiration. We are inundated
by reports of the most beautiful women in the world, who are also in and
out of rehab, in and out of marriages, and snort away a year's wages in
between photo sessions. I don't judge them for any of this: they have been
deceived, their birthright stolen. Their beauty has been defined by a thief,
a thief who hates all women. This enemy conceals the definition of true
beauty, replacing it with a stillborn god that can offer nothing.

God's definition of beauty is vibrant, alive, brilliant, and radiant.
It draws people in. Nothing vibrant is stationary. God's beauty compels
us to action, to give to others. Worldly beauty compels us to consume:
Get attention! Get admiration! Get approval!

Vibrant beauty is the abundant life we're promised, and it prompts
us to seek what we can *give:* give attention, give affirmation, give admiration to others. That's the beauty that leaves its mark on people, and
the world. The thief wants to steal, and God wants to give. When you
contemplate beauty, notice what your definition of beauty is com-
pelling you to do, and you will know who is defining beauty for you at
that moment.

Ask: Pour out Your vibrant beauty into my soul.

Believe: I bless others when I experience God's abundant,
vibrant beauty.

For the temple of God is holy, which temple you are.

—I CORINTHIANS 3:17

When God gave the plans for the temple that King Solomon was to build, no detail was omitted. Every bit of fabrication, color, size, weight, and dimension were articulated. God cared passionately about the place His spirit would dwell. The temple was to become a focal point for the nation, the place where they went to meet God and be ministered to by Him. The temple's intricate, careful design was a way to set this place apart as holy, and to inspire worship of the Designer.

Today, the temple that God indwells is our physical body. However, past religious movements have left their mark on our interpretation of the physical body. We're tempted to denounce it. Ridicule it. Reject it. Flog it. But the truth is, it is the chosen dwelling place of God. If God sees fit to dwell there, who are we to spit at it?

It is no accident that much of our inner battle as women centers on our bodies. We obsess with appearance, weight, and form. The battle over our bodies is really a battle for our souls. We have to choose who we belong to and what we were designed for. If we believe the body is meant for us, then we leave no place for God to inhabit. If we believe our bodies were designed by God as His dwelling place, then we leave no place for worldly judgments about size or "imperfections."

God calls us to recognize the sacred in a world of pollution. Sacred means set apart, not for common use. Something sacred is uncommon and cannot be judged alongside the profane. Sacred also implies it is initiated by God and intended for God. The world's standards are not relevant.

Ask: Teach me what it means to be Your temple.

Believe: I am the delicate, masterful dwelling place of a loving God.

There is no fear in love;
but perfect love casts out fear, because fear involves torment.
—I JOHN 4:18

Perfect means whole and complete. Perfect love can only come from a perfect source. This is the only love that can cast out fear. We cannot free ourselves from fear by thinking around it or avoiding it. We can't even argue or reason with it. Fear has to be cast out by the only thing stronger than itself: perfect love.

Perfect love is stronger than fear because it is whole and complete. Fear is an incomplete revelation. With God, there is no fear without also the hope of complete redemption. The fears that torment us are severed, headless, wingless creatures that can do nothing of consequence without our help. Fear that tortures us is incomplete, because it brings no promise of redemption, no whisper of great hope.

Perfect love is the complete revelation of God. Nothing can stand before its power. It birthed the world and shaped your spirit, and it waits before you today in expectation. Let God's perfect love in, so that it may wipe away the incomplete revelations of Him.

Ask: Reveal Your perfect love to me and cast away my fears.

Believe: God's perfect love is entering my life, and I am whole and complete.

Day Twenty-two: THE PROMISE OF SECURITY

For I am persuaded that neither death nor life,
nor angels nor principalities nor powers, nor things present nor things to come,
nor height nor depth, nor any other created thing,
shall be able to separate us from the love of God which is in Christ Jesus our LORD.

—ROMANS 8:38–39

$\mathcal{T}$he thief whispers to us that physical beauty will give us security. He tells us that beautiful women are loved, wealthy, and immune from life's plagues. Advertisers prey on our craving for security, too, promising we'll be secure if we buy their product and experience, at last, perfect beauty. When we listen to these voices and decide that internal security is based on external appearance, we begin a lifelong dance of frustration and desire.

Just as there is nothing spiritually corrupt in our desire to be called beautiful, there is nothing wrong with our desire for security. We are designed in the core of our being to want, and even crave, security. But what if security comes from within? How would that change us?

Can you envision a bride on her wedding night, that last look in the mirror before walking out of the bathroom and into the bedroom? She makes herself beautiful for the one who had just pledged his life to her. Caring for herself is an expression of love for him. Beauty is rooted in the security of being loved. Beauty doesn't make her feel secure: security makes her feel beautiful.

We are secure. Nothing can separate us from unconditional love. We've been embraced and we are indeed beautiful.

> *Ask:* Let me find security and my soul's peace in You.
> *Believe:* God overturned eternity to prove His love for me.
> I am secure in Him.

23

> *If you take away the yoke from your midst,*
> *The pointing of the finger, and speaking wickedness,*
> *If you extend your soul to the hungry and satisfy the afflicted soul,*
> *Then your light shall dawn in the darkness, and your darkness shall be as the noonday.*
> —ISAIAH 58:9–10

We've all had labels that wounded us: ugly, dumpy, skinny, fat. The wound those labels inflicted was a ragged tear in our souls that ached, and we sought to mend it and soothe the burning shame. We became yoked, chained, to these labels, and daily we dragged our heavy burdens across barren soil that produced nothing but pain in our lives.

I was told I was a monster, that I would never be pretty. The other girls laughed. Boys pointed out my bad teeth and lumpy body. I burned with shame. I wanted to disappear. So I soothed my wound in the silence of isolation.

Finally, one day in school I fled from the teasing and hid in a stairwell with a large skylight. Looking up at God, or at least at the clouds that hid my view of Him, I told Him I would accept being ugly if that was His plan for my life. "But," I added, with all the sincerity that a child has in praying, "if it's all the same to You, I would really rather be beautiful."

Over the next few years, thanks to puberty and braces, my appearance began to change. But the inner wounds didn't heal and I wasn't yet released from my yoke. I needed friends who spoke soothing words, friends who mended what others had torn. Every kind word was a little repair, helping me return to wholeness. My friends were the real answer to my stairwell prayer.

Take every opportunity to speak kindness and encouragement to your sisters today. They are healing too.

Ask: How can I be healed? How can I heal others?

Believe: God is healing me, and I am at peace with myself.

> *The body is a unit, though it is made up of many parts. . . .*
> —I CORINTHIANS 12:12 NIV

Synergy describes the work and intent of God's creation. You could say there is an unfathomable synergy between Father, Son, and Holy Spirit. Everything He has made reflects this synergy: Our bodies have synergy, with many parts that work together. The entire cosmos has synergy, from the planets moving in their orbits around the sun, down to the minute atoms buzzing through the atmosphere.

As we draw near the end of our meditations, we'll soon be considering not only how God created us, but what He gave us in the natural world to accent our well-being and beauty. There is a synergy between God's natural world and the spiritual world. It's a microcosmic reminder of how God intended everything to work in unison for our good: "All things work together for good to those who love God," according to Romans 8:28.

You can't separate the elements of God's multidimensional creation and get optimal results. If you create a physically healthy lifestyle, you must still nurture your spirit. If you want to nurture your spirit, you must care for the body in healthy ways as well. On earth, the spirit needs the body, and the body needs the spirit.

We are all designed to work in unison, as part of the synergy of God's creation, a symphony of women, a blending between the seen and unseen, the logical and the spiritual. Our bodies reflect this balance between the spiritual and physical.

Ask: What physical and spiritual habits do I have that disrupt God's synergy at work in me?

Believe: I will listen to my body *and* my spirit.

And we know that all things work together for good to those who love God,
to those who are the called according to His purpose.

—ROMANS 8:28

God has promised us that everything "works together for good." There is a collective energy in the universe: God's presence. He is pulling everything together and everyone toward Him. The sum of our choices has a collective effect that is greater than any single choice. Any single choice has an impact, but the sum of the choices is exponentially greater. One moment of prayer is great. One act of spiritual obedience is terrific. One healthy meal or one night of deep, restful sleep is wonderful. But a *habit* of any of these will change your life.

God is using everything in your life today to communicate His love for you. Make a habit of allowing His best into your life and heart.

Ask: Help me choose the abundant life in all things.

Believe: My choices work together to bless me.

"Therefore if the Son makes you free, you shall be free indeed."
—JOHN 8:36

*J*esus, who was the essence of beauty, allowed himself to be disfigured so that He could save us. He took the shame of the world upon himself and received it in his body. He set us free. As women who are deeply loved, we are finished with shame and dishonor. Beauty sacrificed himself for us. We cannot buy beauty, but Beauty has bought us. We are redeemed women, ransomed from shame. We can walk proudly because we don't have to exhaust ourselves to find beauty; Beauty found us first and saved us forever.

Ask: Help me to believe in Your death and resurrection.

Believe: Jesus has saved me, and I can anticipate new freedom.

> *Flesh gives birth to flesh, but the Spirit gives birth to spirit.*
> —JOHN 3:6 NIV

What you feed will grow.

If you feed self-doubt, it will grow. If you feed a desire for God's blessings, it will grow.

Every time you make a choice, you move. You move closer to, or further away from, your true self, your true beauty. Making choices that nurture and treat your body with respect will begin to create in you an expectation of honor that will dramatically affect all of your other choices.

In Galatians 5:22–26, the Bible warns us of everything evil we are prone to choose, including contention, jealousy, lewdness, selfish ambition, and jealousy. If we feed this "flesh," or carnal nature, we will become "conceited, provoking one another, envying one another." I recognize this in myself when I compare myself to other women, when I judge a woman as she enters a room. This reaction is from the corrupted nature within, not from God. I can't feed this judgmental nature or it will grow larger and larger until it consumes whatever peace I had when I believed I was loved and called beautiful. It will destroy the harmony I have with other women.

Instead, I have to focus on feeding what needs to grow in my life: true love, for myself and for others, including those women who have what I want or think I need. I am the only one who can water the garden within my spirit where this precious vine grows.

Ask: Give me a fresh encounter with You today.

Believe: I am feeding my beauty, and it is growing.

Blessed are those who hunger and thirst for righteousness,
For they shall be filled.

—MATTHEW 5:6

For He satisfies the longing soul, and fills the hungry soul with goodness.

—PSALM 107:9

$\mathcal{T}$here is a spiritual hunger in the world. I've seen it manifested in an unlikely place: the desire for organic, natural alternatives. Women are tiring of artificial lives and artificial products. We intuitively know something is wrong. We're seeking. There are millions of women who are beginning to explore a "return to nature," an awakening that this artificial concept of beauty may be toxic to us in more ways than one. I've talked to industry leaders, doctors, and researchers for this book, and more than one remarked to me on the growing hunger for "something more."

I think this drive is a reflection of our desire to connect with our Creator. Never before have so many products boasted natural ingredients, essential oils, plant-derived materials, recyclable packaging, and promises that they were not tested on animals.

What we need is not more lotions and creams, but awareness. Awareness of how we're damaging ourselves and how we can be free. Awareness of why we reach for certain products, and what the message is behind each. We need the awareness of God's presence saturating every moment of our lives, and of how utterly loved, completely secure, and beautifully radiant we already are.

Ask: Prepare my heart for the questions You will ask.

Believe: I am beginning an adventure.

❦ 2 ❧

Beauty Secrets: Weight

Women spend billions of dollars trying to achieve the perfect weight, and billions of hours obsessing over it. The first step in achieving the ideal weight is to recognize that the "ideal weight" may be all wrong. Do you know where the American perspective on dieting began, and why? Would it surprise you to learn that our obsession with thinness actually began as a blatant rejection of Christianity?

THE BIRTH OF THE AMERICAN DIET

The Victorian age in America (approximately 1875–1915) was the last age in which Christianity was truly the focal point of American culture. It wasn't perfect. Let me set the stage: Women wore long dresses, even in the summers without air conditioning. Complete modesty ruled the day. People didn't reveal their bodies publicly, so there was much less "body consciousness" in the culture in general. Pornography was not mainstream, so women did not have professional nude models with which to constantly compare their bodies, and cosmetic plastic surgery was still in its infancy.

Men worked and women stayed home, and there was little space for a woman to define herself beyond home and children.

It was even a bit scandalous that men and women had recently begun swimming together in the ocean! Just prior to this, women who wanted to swim "entered the ocean in horse-drawn 'bathing machines,' small, roofless cabins on wheels complete with windows and drapes, where a modest woman could enjoy the healing waters of the sea free from prying male eyes."[1]

Because a woman's place was in the home, bearing children, women were celebrated for having fertile bodies, bodies that were healthy and had generous hips and breasts (assisted by waist-cinching corsets under the clothes). Girls were raised to think only of Christian virtue, not body shape and size. One researcher, the notable Joan Jacobs Brumberg, has spent years comparing the diaries of Victorian girls to modern girls and she concludes that in the Victorian age,

Parents tried to limit their daughters' interest in superficial things, such as hairdos, dresses, or the size of their waists, because character was considered more important than beauty by both parents and the community. And character was built on attention to self-control, service to others and belief in God— not on attention to one's own [body].[2]

Christian morals were the accepted norm, but they were often used wrongly to repress women, to prevent them from becoming full partners in society and marriage. When the women's liberation movement began, one remarkable change occurred: women used their own bodies as a form of protest. They cut off their long, feminine hair. They ditched the long, modest dresses and corsets for straight and short frocks that did not accent full hips or breasts or tiny waists. They taped their breasts flat to their chest. They began drinking, smoking, and being openly sexual. If men had the power and respect of society, women reasoned that they had to become more like men in order to achieve the same privileges. It was the birth of the American flapper, a "revolution in manners and morals."[3]

The first popular American diet book, *Diet & Health, with Key to the Calories* by Lulu Hunt Peters, M.D., was launched in 1918, and obsession with extreme thinness was born. Women were angry, and tired of "Christian morals" that had been used to stifle their contributions. Unfortunately, the rebellion wasn't against the misuse of Christianity, but against Christianity itself. The diet craze of America was rooted in rebellion against God. If you have any doubts about this, consider the practical advice of the Bible: to know what the vine is, look at the fruit it produces (Luke 6:42–44). The obsession with thinness in American has birthed nothing but yo-yo diets, eating disorders, anxiety, and despair.

Today, our focus has shifted from our *behavior* to our *appearance*. More women today are unhappy with their bodies than in the past, and never have we seen such emphasis on improving our bodies and attaining a good life through a good body. It is, researcher Joan Jacobs Brumberg says, "a symptom of historical changes that are only now beginning to be understood."[4]

WHY WE'RE DIFFERENT

The world's leading obesity researchers have discovered that a woman's fat cell is larger than a man's because it has more fat-*storing* enzymes, while a man's fat cell is smaller because it has more fat-*releasing* enzymes. Studies done at Cedars-Sinai Medical Center in Los Angeles and other research facilities have found that a woman's hip and thigh fat cells are at least twice as efficient in storing fat and enlarging as they are in releasing fat and shrinking.[5]

The protesting women of the 1920s got a few things wrong, notably that women are designed to *store* fat. Being thin and boyish, with no hips or breasts, is simply not an achievable, sustainable state for most women, no matter how much tape we use to strap ourselves down. Even thin women still look remarkably feminine and carry more fat in these strategic places than their male counterparts. In chasing the male ideal, women were setting themselves up for a lifetime of failure: a failure that breeds self-contempt, angst, and shame.

There is a wealth of information available about the positive role of fat in our bodies and our cycles, which you can investigate if you feel led. My goal in this chapter is only to introduce the idea to you that you were designed with a very different goal in mind than the male ideal of the protestors. Here is the unavoidable fact: You and I are designed by God to store fat in our hips, stomach, thighs, and breasts. God *wants* us to have fat on our hips, stomach, thighs, and breasts. It was His clear intention.

> God wants *us* to have fat on our hips, stomach, thighs, and breasts. It was His clear intention.

Does it make sense to starve and fight our bodies when they are built to store fat? It seems just as crazy to try to fly by flapping your arms. Your body was designed to store fat, not lose it. Curves are what set you apart from men (that, and the ability to accessorize). Listen to Isaiah 45:9 (MSG): *"But doom to you who fight your Maker—you're a pot at odds with the potter! Does clay talk back to the potter: 'What are you doing? What clumsy fingers!'"*

When we fight our Maker, there's trouble ahead. We've seen that proved time and time again—this obsession with trading in our feminine bodies for male-thin ones has made us fatter, sicker, and more unhappy with ourselves than ever before. Every new generation inherits this curse, as eating disorders continue to claim lives and turn families inside out.

The door that was opened when women rebelled against Christianity was not simply a door to political equality. The door that we opened was one to shame and isolation. We believe there is something wrong with us if we can't shake off those fat cells clinging to our backside and tummy. We don't want others to know that we see something profoundly wrong with our bodies. We resist intimacy, in all its forms and intents. Even our naturally thin sisters suffer in this culture of shame and isolation: they may long for more rounded curves, only to be supported by other women saying things like, "I *hate* you for being so skinny!"

> *Your natural weight is simply defined as the weight you comfortably maintain with a lifestyle of daily exercise and healthy eating.*

To make peace with our weight, we have to make peace with God. We have to make peace with God's design for each unique body. The world may have birthed our ideas about the perfect body image, but it's time for us to do the difficult work of maturing. We can't set the next generation free until we are free. We have to lay down our lives for those we love. We must sacrifice our desire to have the "ideal body" and give up the notion that being beautiful in the eyes of the world will bring us approval and acceptance. If we can do this, we can set our daughters free.

I am not suggesting that obesity is more spiritual than thinness or that thinness is wrong. We're targeting the unhealthy body images and the misery we bring on ourselves in trying to achieve them. Ironically, it's only when we can truly let go of our own unhealthy agendas and preoccupations that we can be free to attend to our health and to achieve a natural weight. Your natural weight is simply defined as the weight you comfortably maintain with a lifestyle of daily exercise and healthy eating.

Queen Esther's Diet

When the king's command and order had been heard, many girls had been brought to the palace in Susa and put under the care of Hegai. . . . Esther pleased Hegai, and he liked her. So Hegai quickly began giving Esther her beauty treatments and special food.
—ESTHER 2:8-9 NCV

When a young girl named Esther was brought into the king's harem and given the chance to win the king's heart to become Queen of the Persian Empire, the first thing her keeper did was put her on a diet! Sounds familiar, you think? In Esther's day, she needed to become pregnant by the king to secure her position in the harem, so this diet was most likely designed to increase her fertility, pad her hips, and spark her desire. I don't think the story of Esther would have ended so well if she had been put on a diet of dry lettuce and clear broth: she'd have been too cranky to woo a king if she was starving!

WHY DIETS ARE UNHEALTHY

Geneen Roth, a writer who specializes in women's food and body issues, once observed, "For every diet, there is an equal and opposite binge."[6] How true! Diets teach us to work against our own bodies, feeding them when they're not hungry with foods they don't want. When we do get hungry, we don't listen to our bodies and either starve ourselves or cram another celery stick down the hatch. Within a few short days, we grow resentful and tired, and then blow the diet. We abandon the produce aisle for the bakery and are never heard from again. That is, until the next reunion or swimsuit season.

The weight-loss industry has fed our mixed emotions with clever marketing and dangerous supplements. They're like the mean girls hanging out in the girls' bathroom. They show us a glimpse of what we can never have, and then promise to give it to us if we'll hand over our lunch money. We feel intimidated, insecure, and we really want to belong, so we hand over the cash. Then our "friends" are nowhere to be found when we're struggling a short time later.

Many researchers have noted the devastating effects this industry has had on women, and one of the most interesting discussions has been about the decline of traditional Christian morals in our culture, and where these morals are reemerging. Morality's new home is in the kitchen. We label foods as bad or good. A recent ad campaign shows a woman who has eaten a donut and shames her with the slogan, "Respect Yourself in the Morning." Just a few decades ago, of course, we all would have understood that slogan to mean, "Don't have immoral, casual sex."

Ironically, we are returning in many ways to the biblical days, labeling healthy foods "clean" and condemning those who eat otherwise. Jesus had to tackle this very doctrine over two thousand years ago. In Matthew 15:10–11 he said,

> *"Hear and understand: Not what goes into the mouth defiles a man; but what comes out of the mouth, this defiles a man."*

There is something in the human soul that longs for the distinction of clean versus unclean, and right versus wrong. Now, overweight women, or even women of normal weight, suspected of eating "unclean" foods, are subjected to the scorn of an invisible scarlet letter *F*. Fat is the new evil. Thin is the new holy. If you have any doubt, flip channels to a diet infomercial: they have all the passion and pathos of an old-time revival.

To make matters worse, women have damaged their health, and even died, from taking over-the-counter diet pills to achieve a thinner body.[7] Except for monitoring labels and advertising, the FDA does not regulate diet pills sold over the counter. If they are proven to be unsafe—which can be a lengthy process—then the FDA can step in and pull them from the market. Every time you pick up a bottle of diet pills, you are placing your life in the hands of strangers. You are betting that they did years of long-term research, that they know how to safely manufacture the ingredients, and that every pill is standardized to contain the exact amount of ingredients listed on the label. But your bet may be wrong.

Thankfully, there is a way out of this danger zone, and into a healthy zone of lasting weight management. You can lose excess weight and learn to love what your body looks and feels like at its natural weight. You can eat the best foods in the world. You can eat until you're deeply satisfied. It shouldn't surprise you by now to know that these secrets have been hidden inside the Bible for centuries.

Why does a person feel full after he or she has eaten? It is not because the stomach is full or because the blood sugar has risen. It depends on the amount one has *smelled* in the process of eating.[8] Smell and taste affect our senses of hunger *and* fullness; taking a moment to savor the aroma of a meal will increase your pleasure in the food, and help curb fast, mindless eating.

Slow down, breathe deeply, and take the time to fully enjoy the food you're blessed with.

THE BEAUTY SECRETS OF THE BIBLE ON WEIGHT

The Bible mentions food thousands of times, either in casual references or in focused moments of teaching. Food was used over and over by Jesus as an illustration, a metaphor for the spiritual world and the inner life. A few years ago I took on an unusual project: I read every reference in the Bible to food, eating, drinking, appearance, and weight. What I learned astonished me:

1. Food is a blessing from God, to be received with thanksgiving.

> *Everything God created is good, and to be received with thanks.* (1 Tim. 4:4 MSG)

> *When you have eaten and are full, then you shall bless the LORD your God for the good land which He has given you.* (Deut. 8:10)

2. Food should taste good: it reminds us of how good God is.

> *Oh, taste and see that the LORD is good.* (Ps. 34:8)

3. Hunger is good, too. It allows us to be empty, so that we can be filled. *"I do not want to send them away hungry,"* Jesus said in Matthew 15:32. The people's hunger was the invitation for one of Jesus' greatest miracles—the feeding of the four thousand.

4. No one is meant to go permanently hungry, but physical hunger can be a temporary teaching tool. Being filled with wonderful food is used as a symbol of God's abundant blessing.

> *So He humbled you, allowed you to hunger, and fed you with*

*manna which you did not know nor did your fathers know,
that He might make you know that man shall not live by bread
alone; but man lives by every word that proceeds from the
mouth of the LORD.* (Deut. 8:3)

*I am the LORD your God, Who brought you up out of the land
of Egypt. Open your mouth wide, and I will fill it.* (Ps. 81:10)

5. Everyone should be able to eat until they are satisfied—not
merely nourished, but *satisfied.*

For he satisfies the thirsty and fills the hungry with good things.
(Ps. 107:9 NIV)

6. You were meant to eat the finest of foods. God's blessing
included good foods, and His ultimate blessing, heaven, is described
as a rich feast.

*He would have fed them also with the finest of wheat; and with
honey from the rock I would have satisfied you.* (Ps. 81:16)

*On this mountain the LORD Almighty will prepare a feast of
rich food for all peoples, a banquet of aged wine—the best of
meats and the finest of wines.* (Isa. 25:6 NIV)

Food is an illustration of the abundance of God. He wants us
to eat our fill. He wants us to have the best. And at the end of our
lives, we can look forward to a feast of supernatural proportions.
Being welcomed into eternal life is repeatedly described in
Scripture as being invited to a wedding feast. We all know the
type of food served at a wedding—rich, delicious, and beautifully presented, with heavenly aromas. We all know how people
eat at a wedding, too: until they are filled and satisfied. Joy and

hope permeate the atmosphere. This is how we were truly meant to live.

7. A proper relationship with food involves making sure others have enough. God's people are commanded to store grain to feed others who have none:

> *The stranger and the fatherless and the widow who are within your gates, may come and eat and be satisfied, that the LORD your God may bless you in all the work of your hand which you do.* (Deut. 14:29)

In a global world, everyone is "within our gates." How are we doing at feeding them, in contrast to ourselves? Consider:

+ America spends $100 billion a year on fast food.[9]
+ Combined, Americans are carrying a total of 7 billion excess pounds on our bodies.[10]
+ Nearly twenty percent of American children go hungry.[11]
+ Six million children die each year, mostly from hunger-related causes, in developing countries.[12]
+ For what Europeans and Americans spend on pet food every year, we could eradicate hunger worldwide.[13]

There is a definite correlation between our wallets and our waists. God has commanded that we care for the physical needs of the poor, making sure everyone has enough to eat. You simply cannot convincingly ask God to bless your weight loss efforts if you are not attending to those who have nothing to eat. Honor God's heart in this matter and see what He is willing to do in yours.

HOW DO I PUT ALL THIS
INTO PRACTICE?

1. Eat when you are hungry. Eat only when hungry. Your body isn't as likely to store food as fat if you eat only when actually hungry.[14] If you eat when you're not hungry, your body doesn't need those calories and will store those calories as fat. When you eat beyond what your body needs, it will throw a fat-storing party: your fat cells can swell to six times their normal size and multiply to store that precious fat.[15]

> *When you eat beyond what your body needs, it will throw a fat-storing party.*

2. Stop eating when satisfied. Satisfied is the point where you stop tasting the food, stop enjoying it, and your mind naturally turns to other things. You're comfortable. Every time you stop when you're satisfied, you are resetting your expectations with food. You're reinforcing the message that you have enough. By not depriving yourself or overindulging, you're creating the expectation in your body that it's okay to let go of excess weight and bad habits.

3. Realize that no one food is off-limits. Diets have done us all a disservice in teaching that certain natural foods are not to be eaten (for example, bananas, or fruits high in carbs). But the truth, according to Pritikin Center nutritionist Dr. Gayl Canfield, is that "The people who eat the most fruit have the most normal weights." Dr. Canfield is known for her work in encouraging people to incorporate many more fruits and vegetables into their diet. She also dispels the idea that certain foods must be eaten in combination. (Some diets teach that foods must be eaten only if paired in specific ways, so that the body can "properly" digest them.) "There's no truth in that," she reassured me.

41

Diets teach us that some foods are "sinful" and not to be eaten. Don't fall for that. If God made it for food, enjoy it. The only foods you should truly avoid are man-made, processed foods, which are loaded with preservatives, refined flours, and trans fats. God has better ones in mind.

God intended for us to eat the "best of the land," which means the foods that will bless and nourish us above all others. Processed foods, loaded with unhealthy ingredients, don't count as the "best of the land" under this definition. They're not "unclean," as some suggest, but you're trading down every time you eat them. How truly generous of God to surround us with natural foods that fight disease and keep us glowing and radiant. If He designed the natural world to silently speak to us of blessing and abundance, how much more would He like to quietly whisper to you as well?

When people eat better, you can tell it on their faces. They feel better. I've seen women beaming. If you improve your internal health, the only possible outcome is that the entire health of the body is improved."
—DR. GAYL CANFIELD

4. Set a daily goal for fruit and vegetable intake. Dr. Wayne Geilman, a nutritional research expert, tells us: "The average American eats only 1.4 servings of fruits and vegetables a day—and that's if you count French fries." He also gave me some startling facts that would send anyone running to the produce aisle:

+ There are 70 diseases linked to the nonconsumption of fruits and vegetables.
+ Over four thousand antioxidants have been identified in fruits and vegetables.

- It has been recently discovered that antioxidants are anti-inflammatory. (Inflammation is suspected as a major cause of premature aging.)
- Consuming these antioxidants will contribute to resilience in your cells, flexibility of membranes, and smoother skin.
- Almost half of what we know about polyphenols (fruit antioxidants) has been discovered only recently. This field of knowledge is rapidly expanding.

We can expect more and more reports of science discovering the potential of fruits and vegetables to unlock the secrets of aging, beauty, and well-being. In the meantime, your body doesn't grade on the curve. Don't compare yourself to your peers—they are only eating 1.4 servings of fruits and vegetables a day, and heart attacks, obesity, cancer, and other diseases are stalking them. You should set a daily goal to eat at least the government's recommendation of six to nine servings per day. Dr. Geilman, however, throws down the gauntlet to us: "Eight to twelve servings a day is better."

5. Never, ever diet again. Studies have shown a clear link between frequent dieting, weight gain, and obesity. One intensive study on the link between yo-yo dieting and increasing percentages of body fat concluded that "going on and off diets repeatedly will make weight control difficult in the long run."[16] Dieting disrupts our naturally beautiful bodies by interfering with our natural appetite cycles, and sets us up for rebellion against healthy foods when we grow tired of trying to diet.

The seduction of diets will be too much for us some days. We'll want to try miracle cures and swear off our favorite foods forever. That's just a natural reaction to living in a diet-saturated media in a processed-food-saturated world. The more you can insulate yourself from diets and weight madness, the more you will:

✤ Discover what your natural weight is (and like it).
✤ Increase your vitality, energy, and well-being.
✤ Appreciate the gift of natural, life-giving foods.

Remember the principle that "What you feed, grows." The more you "feed" this lifestyle, the more it will grow. Health radiates outward, touching every relationship and activity in your life.

BIBLICAL FOODS THAT PROMOTE A HEALTHY WEIGHT

All of the foods below have a strong presence in the Scriptures, and scientists today are only beginning to understand how these foods can benefit our health. But note that *dozens* of different fruits, vegetables, grains, oils, herbs, and spices are mentioned in Scripture. It would take an entire book to examine them all, so we'll highlight only a particular few that can help us find and return to our natural weight.

ALMONDS

Almonds are found throughout Scripture, playing a role in our diet as well as in God's message to us. The Hebrew word for almonds means "diligence," and the flowers of the almond plant symbolize the awakening of spring.[17] The beautiful plant suggests the new spring we will someday be led into, the spring of freedom and redemption from slavery, poverty, and war, an awakening of spirit and heart.

In Jeremiah 1:10–11, God shows Jeremiah an almond tree,

known as a *šōqēd*. This is meant to symbolize God's *šōqēd*, or "watching," and gives evidence of God's commitment to fulfill His prophecy: "for I am ready to perform My word" (Jer. 1:10–12).[18]

Modern science backs up the idea that almonds are little blessings: not only do almonds have a role in significantly reducing bad cholesterol, they may also help you lose weight and improve metabolic syndromes.[19] That means almonds may play a role in helping our bodies use insulin efficiently and shed excess, harmful weight.

Setting bowls of fresh fruit and nuts (especially nuts in the shell) around your home not only looks inviting, but it encourages healthy snacking. Having these foods nestled in attractive bowls throughout your home sends a message of abundance.

The recommended dose of these little treasures is approximately one ounce, or ¼ cup, per day. You can find a fabulous recipe for a snack mix using these on page 84. Raw almonds with brown skins are the best kind to use. Commercially roasted nuts contain added fats and will go bad faster than raw nuts.

Almonds Are All-That

+ Almond skins contain more than 20 antioxidants. [20]
+ These antioxidants combine with the vitamin E found inside the almond's meat to deliver more than double the power of antioxidants than if they were consumed alone. [21]
+ Consuming whole, raw almonds in a heart-healthy diet

can lower damaging inflammation levels as well as statin drugs. [22]

❖ Eating almonds as part of a healthy diet can help you lose 62 percent more weight than a diet without almonds, plus achieve a 50 percent greater reduction in waist size and 56 percent greater reduction in body fat. [23]

❖ Oh, yes—and thanks to the vitamin E they contain, almonds are a wonderful food for fighting premature aging and wrinkles!

FLAX

In biblical times, flax, and especially flax oil, was used for making linen and for food, and the flaxseed was valued for its medicinal properties. Flax also was featured in two epic biblical tales: God destroyed the flax crops of the Egyptians in the Seventh Plague (Exod. 9:31), and Rahab used stalks of flax to hide the spies, Joshua and Caleb, on her roof (Josh. 2:6).

Today, researchers believe the omega-3 fatty acids in flax help the body regulate leptin, which helps you lose weight and burn fat more efficiently. Omega-3s are also important as anti-inflammatory agents, and according to *First* magazine, flax is "nature's number one source of lignans, unique plant compounds that can double the speed at which the liver metabolizes and excretes inflammation-triggering fat and toxins. The study-proven dose: 1 to 2 Tbs. of ground flax daily."[24] Because ground flaxseed is so rich in fiber, it can help keep your blood sugar stable and help you avoid low-blood-sugar munchies. For maximum benefit and taste, buy a coffee grinder and whole flaxseeds, and grind a little fresh every morning to add onto your cereal, toast, or breakfast shake.

You've probably seen ads for diet pills that promise to optimize your leptin levels. These over-the-counter pills can take a bite out of your wallet.

Cost for 30-day supply of "leptin" diet pills: $99

Cost for 30-day supply of flaxseed: $5

TOTAL SAVINGS: $1,128 per year (based on buying one bag of flaxseeds per month versus one bottle of diet pills per month)

Besides saving you money, flax offers advantages no diet pill can offer:

- ❖ Flax has six times the fiber of oatmeal.
- ❖ Flax is higher in lignans, which protect us from disease, than any other source. One-fourth cup ground flaxseed has more lignans than 60 cups of broccoli.
- ❖ Flax can be substituted for butter in many baked goods. Cut the amount of butter called for in half, and use this same amount of ground flax in its place.

FISH

Fish and fishing were a biblical way of life and a staple of the everyday diet. They were roasted fresh, or dried to be eaten later. Several of the Bible's disciples were fishermen before they met Jesus, including Peter, Andrew, James, and John. Jesus even performed miracles with fish, feeding multitudes of hungry followers and providing the disciples with a miraculous catch of fish.

*E*verything works together for good:

Fish high in omega-3s are not only good for achieving a healthy weight and preventing premature aging, but studies have now linked consumption of omega-3s with a reduction in depression.[25] Only God can create natural foods that bless us in so many ways.

All fish are a good source of protein. Some fish are also a rich source of omega-3s, which not only can help you lose excess weight, but also contribute to healthy, soft skin. It's always best to eat whole foods instead of supplements, but because of concerns over high mercury levels in some types of fish, I mix both supplements and servings of fish into my routine. If you use a supplement, buy one that promises no fishy aftertaste.

CINNAMON

Cinnamon was used in the holy anointing oil for the tabernacle, a prophetic symbol of the Holy Spirit's anointment on our lives. Modern research tells us that cinnamon plays a role in regulating blood sugar. By adding cinnamon supplements to your diet each day you may help boost your glucose metabolism, prevent blood sugar spikes, improve cholesterol levels, and help your body return to its natural weight.[26] Look for cinnamon supplements, which are simply powdered cinnamon packaged inside gel capsules; the proven dosage is the equivalent of 1/4 to 1/2 teaspoon daily. Supplements are a convenient way to get your cinnamon each day, and are quite inexpensive. Cinnamon sprinkled on your food may not be as beneficial, since saliva contains a chemical harmful to cinnamon.[27]

> ## Type 3 Diabetes
>
> There may be a connection between high blood sugar, inflammation, and Alzheimer's, which some are now referring to as a possible "type 3" diabetes.[28] Taking steps to ensure stable blood sugar, such as by consuming cinnamon and flax, may play an important role in reducing your risk of such diseases.

CLOVES

Cloves get their name from the Latin word *clavus*, meaning "nail," because they look very much like nails. Because spices were so valuable in biblical days, they were kept in a king's treasury. Second Kings 20:13 tells of King Hezekiah showing off "all the house of his treasures—the silver and gold, the spices and precious ointment, and all in his armory—all what was found among his treasures." A life-giving spice that is undervalued in our culture, cloves, like cinnamon, may play an important role in regulating glucose levels, lowering cholesterol—especially the bad type—and helping to reduce weight and promote lean body mass.[29] They make beautiful additions to many dishes. You can add them into your favorite tea, or mix into a fruit vinaigrette. I love the smell of cloves so much I throw a few into a candle and allow the melted wax to warm and release their scent.

FIGS

The fig tree symbolizes prosperity and peace in Micah 4:4: "Everyone shall sit under his vine and under his fig tree, and no one shall make them afraid."[30] We've discovered that figs, because they are rich in fiber, can help promote a return to a normal weight. They also are helpful in protecting bone density and protecting the cardiovascular system.[31] Dried figs are available year-round but lack the fiber of fresh figs. Because heart disease is the number one killer of women, and we struggle with osteoporosis as well, figs may be a rich blessing to us indeed.

VINEGAR

Vinegar was as common as wine in biblical days, and different varieties were made by the addition of herbs. Vinegar has been in the news lately for its suspected ability to slow carbohydrate absorption and encourage stable blood sugar. Dr. Carol Johnston of Arizona State University East of Mesa has published research that demonstrates consuming two tablespoons of vinegar before a meal prevents the blood sugar spikes that come from eating carbohydrates. The effect is comparable to antidiabetes drugs, and is most effective for those who are showing signs of becoming diabetic.[32] Participants in Dr. Johnston's study also lost a modest amount of weight, between two to four pounds in four weeks when consuming two tablespoons of vinegar twice daily before meals.

I asked Dr. Johnston if any vinegar might be substituted for the vinegar used in the study (which was apple cider vinegar). Participants didn't like the taste of drinking the apple cider vinegar, but since the suspected active ingredient studied, acetic acid, is present in all vinegars, Dr. Johnston confirmed that mine was, indeed, a reasonable conclusion, and is in fact doing studies now with red raspberry vinegar.

A word of caution: don't buy vinegar pills. They may not contain acetic acid, the active ingredient studied. Dr. Johnston is working on creating a supplement that does contain acetic acid, so save your money until she does.

BREAD

Bread was the mainstay of the biblical diet. The words *bread* and *food* were interchangeable. Bread was made from either wheat or barley, and the women ground the grains and baked the bread fresh each day, except for the Sabbath.

Bread plays an important role in how we understand our dependence on God, and His nature. In the wilderness, the Israelites depended on God to provide manna, which had to be gathered fresh each day. When Jesus arrived, he said this about Himself: "I am the bread of life. He who comes to me shall never hunger." (John 6:35).

Manna was a foreshadowing of Christ, the Word dwelling among us from heaven. This dependence on God for spiritual nourishment as well as physical is taught throughout Scripture.

> *But He answered and said, "It is written, 'Man shall not live by bread alone, but by every word that proceeds from the mouth of God.'"* (Matt. 4:4)

> *Give us this day our daily bread.* (Matt. 6:11)

*A*ll breads are not equal. Making *whole grains* a focus of your diet will help reduce your risk of disease, keep you feeling full longer, and help stabilize blood sugar.

BEAUTY SECRETS OF THE BIBLE (BSB) RECIPES

ALMOND-FILLED SWEET POTATO

Here's a snack that multitasks: it helps you achieve a natural weight, encourages glowing skin with fewer premature wrinkles, and lowers bad cholesterol. Sweet potatoes do not cause the same rise in blood sugar that white potatoes do.

Steam one large sweet potato by pricking with a fork and microwaving until soft to the touch. Add in raw almonds, chopped, and cinnamon to taste.

You'll fill up on ingredients that promote a return to your natural weight, plus promote smooth and radiant skin.

BSB CHOCOLATE CHIP FLAXSEED COOKIES

We've already seen that ground flaxseed helps women with problems such as dandruff, dry skin, and premature aging. But how to work flax into the diet? I sprinkle it on my breakfast cereal and into my baked goods. One recipe is a classic at my house: Chocolate Chip Flaxseed Cookies.

Dark chocolate in moderation can be good for you, and these cookies are a healthy way to indulge. Each cookie has more healthy lignans (antioxidants that promote breast and colon health) than ten cups of broccoli! Each cookie also packs a powerful punch of fiber that will keep you full and satisfied, promoting weight loss. There's no cholesterol, and the cookies may even promote heart health and a healthier cholesterol level. Chocolate never was so good, and good for you!

BSB CHOCOLATE CHIP FLAXSEED COOKIES

½   cup heart-healthy butter substitute
½   cup ground flaxseeds
¾   cup natural brown sugar

½   cup unbleached granulated sugar
1   egg
1   tablespoon vanilla extract
1   cup whole wheat flour
1 ¼ cups unbleached all-purpose flour
½   teaspoon salt
1   teaspoon baking soda
1   12-ounce package dark chocolate chips

First, cream butter, flaxseeds, and sugars until well mixed. Add egg and vanilla. In a separate bowl, combine flours, salt, and soda. Mix thoroughly and stir into wet ingredients. Add chocolate chips.

Drop onto cookie sheet using a medium-sized melon baller or large spoon. Bake at 375 degrees for 10 minutes. Makes 22 large cookies.

Indulge Me

*T*ea isn't mentioned in the Bible. However, we know the people in biblical times were trading with the East. Many of the biblical wars were fought for control of the trade routes, which brought them in contact with those as far away as Africa and India. These same trade routes also helped spread the gospel later.

So it is possible the earlier biblical peoples knew about tea. Tea is, of course, one of God's most notable health foods. Not only does tea fight free radicals, cancer, and give us a soothing, nurturing moment of rest, it can also help us lose weight. Green tea in particular has been studied for its ability to boost metabolism and burn fat. But skip the supplements and drink it fresh. Keep it iced to sip on throughout the day, and don't forget to fill a small spritzer to place in the fridge as a wrinkle-fighting facial spritz. (A spritzer with freshly brewed tea should be refilled at least weekly to keep tea fresh.) Tea's magic is in its catechin polyphenols and flavonoids, "anti-inflammatory compounds that are 200 times more powerful than even vitamin E at soothing cellular inflammation."[33] When drinking tea, make it even more powerful by adding a few cloves while it steams, and swirl a cinnamon stick into it for a beautiful presentation. If you have trouble with snacking at night, establish a new routine of drinking herb tea after dinner instead of eating.

WHY EXERCISE?

I want you to consider *why* you exercise. That reason is probably the number one reason you quit, too. Do you exercise because you're fat and need to lose weight? Do you visualize yourself getting smaller and thinner? Do you get disgusted with the minuscule progress you make and quit? I believe the motivation that gets us to work out can ultimately be our undoing.

Think about the dynamics of life. What is the strongest instinct any creature has? It's the will to live. When you send messages to the body that it must become smaller, give up food, and get rid of stored fat, you're sending it messages that it may interpret as a threat to its survival. No creature is wired to desire becoming less. We are all wired to want more. (I believe that's what got us into this mess!)

Sending yourself the right message can change your life, not just your weight. Focus on eating *more:* especially *more* fruits and *more* vegetables, as well as more whole grains and lean sources of protein and dairy. Focus on exercising to build yourself up, to get *more*—more endurance and more muscle.

STRENGTH

There's a difference between fat-burning aerobic exercise that builds endurance, and muscle-creating exercise that builds strength. A lot of women concentrate on aerobic exercise and miss half of the exercise equation. Muscle-building exercises—specifically, training with weights—will decrease your size while building muscle. Weight training is a critical workout regimen that many of us may be missing.

There is an integrity we discover when we *build* our bodies. The action of working out to build it, to get more life for it, sends the subliminal message that your body is already at a good starting point. It's a message of acceptance, a belief you already have something of worth and worth building upon. This focus automatically eliminates comparison to others: it's a dramatic process of affirming yourself even as you work to build upon what you have.

Anytime we can switch the focus from what we look like to what we actually do, we line ourselves up spiritually with every doctrine in the Scriptures. The abundant life isn't about appearance. It's about how our new life is manifested in what we do. It's about reaching out for more, instead of believing the lies that lead to shame and isolation.

A HISTORY OF WEAK WOMEN

If you're feeling a bit skittish about working out with weights, I have an insight that might shock you. God intended for you to be strong:

> *She girds herself with strength, and strengthens her arms.*
> (Prov. 31:17)

Think about our biblical sisters. They had to walk in the desert for forty years, lugging babies and household supplies. They had to draw water and carry the heavy pitchers back to their homes, every day. They had to grind their own grains. A strong woman survived and her family thrived. Strength in women has always been prized throughout history, anytime in a culture that people lived close to the land, including the early days of America. When the Industrial Revolution hit, women didn't need to do all of those tasks. We could buy ground flour. We could buy produce, and soap, and clothes. It was during this shift in our habits, from strong worker to the modern consumer, that the "weak woman" came into vogue. Femininity was redefined as weakness.

Suddenly, strong women weren't necessarily valuable women. Men, especially wealthy men, didn't have to choose wives based on how strong and capable they were. About this time, fainting couches came into style, and the myth of the weak woman was born. We became luxury items—a rich man could afford a woman who was so weak she couldn't get off the couch. We became trophy wives instead of capable, strong partners.

Women were meant to be strong. Don't fall for the lingering lie that deliberately weak women are more feminine. Your strength, in every way, only enhances and accents a man's strength.

THE WISDOM OF CELEBRATING EACH OTHER

One of the greatest blessings of diversity, which is God's intended order of life, is that as diverse women enter the pages of magazines and are on television and in movies, we are seeing a celebration of body types that extend well beyond what American writer Tom Wolfe once called the "impeccably emaciated" ideal. Every action has unexpected effects. No one knew that pushing our culture to embrace more than one standard of beauty would begin to relieve all women of the burdens of isolation and condemnation. Praise God for making us all so different, and for those on earth who have the wisdom to celebrate that!

May you, too, be continually blessed as you search for balance between spirit and beauty, strength and gentleness, wisdom and application. I pray that the changes you make as you continue the *Beauty Secrets of the Bible* journey will create changes in every area of your life, bringing health and joy to you and yours.

❦ 3 ❦

Beauty Secrets the Cosmetic Industry Doesn't Want You to Know

W e're moving on now to the routines we go through every morning when we prepare for our day. Many of us never consider the products we use, what they're made with, and how they might be affecting our lives. We've seen that when God creates something, it blesses us in many ways. But when humans get busy in a laboratory, anything can happen. Some of the products you are using may be undoing what you're trying to do by reading this book and embracing a new, healthier view of beauty. Some of the products you're using may be harming your body, and sending quiet messages that undermine His affirming love for you just as you are.

There are secrets lurking in your bathroom. Every day, you're slathering yourself in products that have been linked to breast cancer, fertility problems, hormone disruptions, and other assorted ailments. They're made from slaughterhouse waste and chemicals that are also found in engine degreasers, metal polish, and toilet bowl cleaner. And you paid top dollar for them.

"What?" you ask. "Everything I buy is straight off the shelf at my local drugstore or department store. It's safe. It's from well-known companies."

Hold onto your hand cream, ladies. I am about to reveal the secrets that the cosmetic industry may not want you to know.

Let's begin with a pop quiz. What does this list have in common?

Turtle oil
Chicken embryo
Horse blood
Pigskin
Human placenta
Pig brains
Cow amniotic fluid

According to the FDA, these are raw materials actually used in certain beauty products.[1] The FDA states, "A cosmetic manufacturer may essentially use any raw material in a product and market it without prior FDA approval."[2]

Are you sure you know what's in your bathroom cabinets?

SECRETS ABOUT THE FDA

The FDA does not regulate the cosmetic industry as we expect it would. Beauty care companies do not have to prove a product is safe before putting it on the market. They don't have to get approval for using pig brains and selling it to you as a new miracle treatment, guaranteed to prevent wrinkles, eliminate cellulite, and perk up breasts. In fact, they don't even have to tell you the truth. The FDA also admits that "cosmetic claims, even those considered 'puffery,' are allowed without scientific substantiation."[3]

It's bad enough that we're being misled and lied to so we'll use products that may not work. It's bad enough we're being sold products that began as industrial waste. But even worse, some of these products may have health risks. Here is the final blow against our assumption of protection: only 11 percent of cosmetic ingredients have been assessed for safety by the cosmetic industry.[4]

> Only 11 percent of cosmetic ingredients have been assessed for safety by the cosmetic industry.

So to sum up the state of the industry, a beauty products company can put almost anything in a product, make almost any false claim they want, and sell it to you for an exorbitant price. And it's all legal.

But how risky is it to use a face cream with a minor amount of a potential toxin? Perhaps the risk is indeed very minute. But we don't just use face cream, do we? We use cleanser, moisturizers, creams, anti-wrinkle lotions, sunscreens, body lotions, deodorants, hair mousse, hairspray, and lip plumpers. This is all *before* we begin to apply our cosmetics! One tiny amount of an ingredient perhaps would not be so troublesome, but we use much more than one product a day. The Campaign for Safe Cosmetics sums up the situation nicely:

> *The chemicals in any one consumer product alone are unlikely to cause harm. But unfortunately, we are repeatedly exposed to industrial chemicals from many different sources on a daily basis, including cosmetics and personal care products. Some of these chemicals are linked to cancer, birth defects and other health problems that are on the rise in the human population. Some chemicals found in a variety of cosmetics—including phthalates, acrylamide, formaldehyde and ethylene oxide—are listed by EPA and the state of California as carcinogens or reproductive toxins. Major loopholes in federal law allow the $35 billion cosmetics industry to put unlimited amounts of chemicals*

into personal care products with no required testing, no monitoring of health effects, and inadequate labeling requirements. [5]

Could our constant exposure to these chemicals be behind some of the health conditions that plague us? Are we unwittingly increasing our risk of breast cancer and other ailments? Consider this:

Over the years there has been a steady rise in women's health conditions such as breast cancer, fibroids, endometriosis, miscarriage, and infertility. There also has been a rise in conditions such as fibromyalgia, chronic fatigue syndrome and hypothyroidism, which mostly affect women. Studies show that human exposure to chemicals in our environment such as pesticides, herbicides, insecticides, and manufacturing byproducts, can cause these endocrine disrupting conditions. [6]

According to the FDA, only eight ingredients are banned from cosmetics in the United States. The European Union has banned more than 1,000. Industry expert Kathryn Higgins encourages us that "we all need to become educated on the health effects of ingredients in our cosmetics and household products because we can't assume the cosmetic industry and government agencies are doing this for us."

WHAT TO WATCH FOR

Let's take a closer look at a handful of beauty product chemicals suspected as dangerous to our health, and you can begin screening your beauty products for these ingredients.

PARABENS

A preservative used in almost all beauty products, parabens have been linked to breast cancer. Parabens have been found in breast cancer tumors.[7] It is still unclear whether parabens simply accumulate in tumors or actually incite tumor growth.

While there is a raging debate over whether parabens are safe, one fact is clear: parabens, which are petroleum by-products, have the ability to accumulate in human tissue. You can expect a number of studies to appear in the next few years on the issue, but for now, it does seem wise to limit your exposure to parabens whenever possible.

> The irony is, every time I did a monthly breast self-exam, I stepped out of the shower and slathered on a body lotion that was potentially increasing my risk of breast cancer.

To show you just how pervasive these parabens are, I challenge you to check the products in your bathroom. If you see any ingredient that ends in the word *paraben,* you've been exposed. I checked my cabinets and found a total of eleven products with parabens. The irony is, every time I did a monthly breast self-exam, I stepped out of the shower and slathered on a body lotion that was potentially increasing my risk of breast cancer.

Remember, parabens are used almost universally in beauty products: More than 13,000 products registered with the American Food and Drug Administration contain parabens. A survey of 215 cosmetics found that 99 per cent of those designed to be left on the skin contained parabens.[8]

Parabens are cheap. They make cosmetics more affordable and prevent bacteria from growing in your product. They prolong the long shelf life that keeps costs down for manufacturers and consumers alike. There are alternatives, such as a few fruit-based preservatives on the market, but these are expensive to manufacture and can drive a product's cost out of reach for some consumers.

If manufacturers could cheaply swap out parabens for another preservative, they probably would. However, as one industry insider told me, you can't swap one preservative for another. Changing the preservative affects everything about a product, including the color and feel. It's going to be a financial catastrophe for manufacturers if parabens are proven to be unsafe. Almost every product on the market will have to be reformulated, at an enormous cost. In the next chapter, I'll show you some luxurious switches you can make that will limit your exposure to parabens.

DEA

The National Toxicology Program found an association between the cosmetic ingredient DEA (and DEA-related ingredients) when topically applied and cancer in laboratory animals.[9] DEA is diethanolamine. A closely related chemical is TEA, or triethanolamine.

PHTHALATES

A Harvard study has linked phthalates with damage to sperm.[10] This may, in turn, increase male infertility rates and birth defects.[11] You may have seen labels on children's toys promising to be "phthalate free." The scare was significant enough to prompt manufacturers to get rid of any phthalates in toys that could be chewed on or handled by babies. However, the cosmetic industry continues to put them in products that adults, including women of child-bearing age, use daily, and the CDC has reported elevated levels of phthalates excreted in the urine of women of child-bearing age.[12]

Phthalates include dibutylphthalate (DBP), dimethylphthalate (DMP), and diethyl phthalate (DEP). Because these can be used in fragrance, and fragrances don't have to list the individual components, these toxins are not always easy to detect on a cosmetic label—you must resort to calling the manufacturer or checking the Campaign for Safe Cosmetics database. A website for this database is included in the Resource Guide.

OTHER POTENTIAL TOXINS WORTH MENTIONING

Other potential toxins may be used in products. Recently, a cellulite cream was introduced to the market that contains esculin. Esculin, according to the Mayo Center, is "associated with significant toxicity and death."[13] But of course, the manufacturer is under no obligation to conduct safety testing prior to selling the product, and consumers don't know if applying this toxin to this skin will produce health risks similar to those as ingested.

Two other ingredients in particular are the subject of much debate. Some feel they have hidden health hazards, but they are widely used in the cosmetic industry and believed by many experts to be safe. Still, you may want to be aware of them:

1. *Sodium lauryl sulfate.* This is a detergent used in shampoos and soaps. It can be harsh and can cause irritated skin and a flaking or irritated scalp. However, it is inexpensive and therefore attractive for manufacturers. Almost every shampoo and body wash I checked at retail contained it. If you struggle with dry or irritated skin, a wise step would be to seek out alternative products. I recently bought a famous-brand bath soap that promised to be "detergent free." To my surprise, sodium lauryl sulfate was the major ingredient listed. But since it's legal to mislead consumers, I shouldn't have been surprised. (As a special note, if you are African-American or Hispanic, your skin may be especially sensitive to irritation from this ingredient.[14])

2. *Petroleum.* Petroleum and petroleum products (mineral oil, petrolatum, petroleum) are used in many cosmetic preparations,

and there is a lingering debate over whether petroleum products are completely safe or effective. Advocates for banning petroleum say it does not allow skin cell turnover and increases premature aging, and that contaminants from the manufacturing process can cause a health risk.

The scientific community has determined that petroleum is, however, an effective barrier moisturizer: that is, it forms a barrier that does not release moisture from the skin and protects it from the elements. You should consider where petroleum comes from, how it is made, and decide whether switching to another body oil would make sense for you: Unrefined petroleum contains natural gas, gasoline, benzene, kerosene, diesel fuel, and tars. During the refining process, the differing weights between the components separate themselves out and manufacturers create the different final petroleum products, including refined petroleum for use in medicine and personal care. [15] Much of the debate about petroleum's safety for our skin centers around this process, because it is suspected that toxic contaminants can hitch their way into the petroleum.

While the debate rages on, my own pediatrician warned me against using petroleum-based products on my daughter, who suffers from eczema, specifically telling us to avoid baby oil. His opinion is that baby oil, because it is based on mineral oil, dries skin out more than it replenishes it. I have experienced this myself, and perhaps you have too. Have you applied a moisturizer and about an hour later, felt your skin was dry again? Thankfully God has supplied some amazing natural moisturizers that nourish your skin, heal it, and have been well-studied and proven to work. They're minimally processed, packed with antioxidants, and much less expensive than commercial moisturizers. (I'll give you more details in a later chapter and tell you where you can purchase the oils.)

CHEMICALS DOING DOUBLE DUTY

Even in familiar, trusted brands, we simply don't know what we're really using. The simplest of products can contain an enormous number of chemicals. These chemicals aren't just used in cosmetics, either—they have double lives. My former "gentle" eye makeup remover contains chemicals also found in antifreeze, pesticide, toilet bowl cleaner, furniture stripper, tire cleaner, and gas treatments.

> My former "gentle" eye makeup remover contains chemicals also found in antifreeze, pesticide, toilet bowl cleaner, furniture stripper, tire cleaner, and gas treatments.

My former favorite daytime moisturizer, which promised to regenerate my skin's appearance, contains chemicals also used in battery cleaner, color-safe bleach, Pine-Sol®, concrete primer, and metal polish.

The more you know about what you're buying, the less pretty you feel. The problem isn't chemicals—after all, you could say *we're* made of chemicals—but the problem is with synthetic chemicals that may be affecting us in ways we don't yet understand.

THE GROSS-OUT FACTOR

Have you ever bought a lipstick or skin cream that promised it was enriched with collagen? Sounds lovely, doesn't it? Maybe, until you learn that collagen can be manufactured from slaughterhouse waste. Sources for collagen include pigskin, cowskin, and, in the case of "marine collagen," fish scales.

Ingredients manufactured from slaughterhouse waste may include:

Tallow

Oleic acid

Glycerin
Collagen
Keratin
Gelatin

There are currently twenty-five facilities in the United States that convert slaughterhouse waste into raw materials for cosmetics.[16] But getting information about the waste is difficult at best. If you see any of these ingredients on the label, you won't know if they came from slaughterhouse waste or were synthetically created. Many of the manufacturers don't even know. The companies that supply raw materials to the company may not divulge that information. Your best bet is to look for labels that say "No Animal By-Products," or "100 Percent Vegan."

KEEP IN MIND

Whatever you apply on the skin can be absorbed into the body. Nicotine and birth control patches work on this principle. Applying beauty products may allow any ingredient to be absorbed into the skin and into the bloodstream. Many beauty products are specifically engineered to penetrate the skin's barrier to deliver the chemicals and create "results."

We just don't know what effects these products have, long-term. But testing would require millions of dollars, and time, which beauty care companies simply don't have in an age that thrives on introducing a new product every few months.

"BUT I USE ALL-NATURAL PRODUCTS"

That's what you think.

But just because a label says the word *natural*, don't assume it's good for your skin. Wil Baker, an organics expert, told me, "The word 'natural' on a label is virtually meaningless." Another industry expert, organic chemist Kimberly Sayer, echoes this. "The FDA allows a product to be labeled legally as 'natural' if only 3 percent of the ingredients are natural." That other 97 percent of ingredients may, in fact, be synthetic chemicals, including petroleum waste products.

There are many companies today that aggressively market products as natural that are using paraben preservatives, petroleum by-products, and other noxious ingredients.

Other "meaningless" terms on beauty products include:

Organic: There are no federal regulations for what constitutes an "organic" cosmetic. "Organic" beauty products may in fact be loaded with synthetic chemicals.

Alcohol free: According to the FDA, this "traditionally means [the products] do not contain ethyl alcohol (or grain alcohol). Cosmetics products, however, may contain other alcohols, such as cetyl, stearyl, cetearyl, or lanolin." [17]

Fragrance free: The FDA says this "implies that [the product] has no perceptible odor. Fragrance ingredients may be added to a fragrance-free cosmetic to mask any offensive odor." [18]

Hypo-allergenic: This implies certain ingredients known for causing negative reactions are not present. There are no federal standards for this term and companies may use it as they please.

Dermatologist-tested: A dermatologist most likely did patch tests on human skin to see if the product caused a reaction. It doesn't mean the product is free of chemicals that may cause long-term health concerns.

Pediatrician or dermatologist recommended: In some cases, a doctor was paid to endorse a product.

"BUT ORGANICS COMPANIES USE
PRESERVATIVES TOO"

Of course they do: milk left on the kitchen counter spoils, and so do many natural ingredients. Preservatives aren't the enemy, and neither are chemicals. What we should object to is any ingredient with known health issues. There are natural products that don't require preservatives, and there are natural preservative systems available to manufacturers.

As you begin this journey, you may not want to change everything in your routine. That's okay. I haven't, either. Going natural for one product does not obligate you to go natural with every product. Often, however, seeing a difference in your appearance will make you curious enough to try more, but that's the fun of the journey.

Women haven't been taught to read beauty labels . . . until now. I predict that a label revolution is going to take place in America: just as women have been taught how to read food labels and make wise choices, women will begin to look more closely at the ingredients of their beauty products. Knowledge is power.

A few years ago, trans fats were in thousands of grocery items. Scientists knew how dangerous these were to our health, but they were cheap fats with long shelf life, so the food industry kept using them. As the public educated themselves, demand for products that were "trans fat free" began to capture the attention of manufacturers. If they wanted to sell their products, they had to remove the trans fats. Today, the companies must clearly label the amount of trans fat in every product, and many products boast that they are trans fat free. Companies didn't make the switch because these fats were bad for us— they made the switch because they risked losing business.

When women are given the knowledge of what they're buying, they make different decisions, and the industry responds.

BEAUTIFUL, NATURALLY

We're spending billions of dollars a year on products that are potentially harmful and make unsubstantiated claims. That's money we can all use in better ways. In this book, I'll teach you how to replace hundreds of dollars' worth of commercial products with ancient remedies that really work. These products are backed up with scientific studies and are safe, natural, and healthy. In fact, these products are so healthy, doctors even recommend eating many of them every day! (When's the last time you found a recipe on the back of your drugstore moisturizer?)

Every woman deserves to feel beautiful, no matter how much money is in her wallet, and no matter what the magazines say. Oddly, many of us would understand the need to throw out a Ouija board or a pornographic magazine. We understand how those objects contaminate a life. But have we ever considered how beauty products are souring our spirits? When they're sold by creating doubts about our desirability, about our worth and appearance, they're trespassing on our inheritance. In their world, aging is to be avoided at all costs, fat is the enemy, and beauty is just a commodity. Any ingredient is acceptable as long as it promises beauty. Every time you pick up that package, whether you are conscious of it or not, you're reinforcing that message internally. That's another great reason to consider incorporating more natural beauty alternatives into your regimen.

We're paying high prices for advertising and marketing. Natural products that we feature in this book don't have ad campaigns with the mega-wattage of an international cosmetic company. But starting today, you're going to be spending your money on *product*, not *promotion*. No ad ever improved your skin. No television commercial ever prevented a single wrinkle. Don't waste your money on what will never reach your skin.

Besides, God doesn't need a slick ad campaign. He's already got one, and it runs 24/7:

> *The heavens declare the glory of God;*
> *the skies proclaim the work of his hands;*
> *Day after day they pour forth speech;*
> *night after night they display knowledge.* (Ps. 19:1–2 NIV)

Who can top what God has created? I checked the label of my former favorite body lotion (one that had been potentially exposing me to the risk of breast cancer), and it had no less than thirty ingredients, all formulated to try and achieve a lasting feeling of moisture when applied to the skin. In the next chapter, I'm going to show you a natural moisturizer that is simply amazing—and it has exactly one ingredient. No matter how many hours scientists spend in a lab, there's just nothing better than God's handiwork.

❧ 4 ❧

Beauty Secrets: Skin

When our skin looks good, we feel radiant—and need fewer cosmetics. Skin care products are designed to be applied and left on the skin, so it's important to use the healthiest products possible. I'm going to give you a three-step regimen that focuses on facial care, but all of the products can be used on the body for great results, too. This regimen can be followed morning, night, or both.

All of the products we'll discuss should be available at your local grocer and are inexpensive, pleasing alternatives to commercial products. I recommend you begin by making a small investment in some containers, spritz bottles, and cosmetic jars. How we feel about what we're using is as important as the ingredients themselves. Biblical women knew this—many archeological finds have been elaborate cosmetic containers, carved out of exquisite ivories and stone, and fashioned into fantastical shapes such as ornate lions, with the bowl grasped between the fierce paws, or women swimming with their arms outstretched. Women want to feel good about what we're using, and the packaging matters.

In the Resource Guide, I'll show you how to buy wholesale cosmetic packaging—the same packaging that the cosmetic industry uses. Or, you can visit a giant retailer like Wal-Mart and buy small containers in the travel-sized sample area. Either way, you'll be creating the most exclusive line of beauty products on earth—custom tailored for your unique needs.

*I*n the Bible, one of the most common shapes for body oil containers was a horn. In I Samuel 16:13, it is with such a horn that Samuel anoints a young David as king of Israel:

Then Samuel took the horn of oil and anointed him in the midst of his brothers; and the Spirit of the LORD came upon David from that day forward.

STEP ONE: WASH AND EXFOLIATE

My favorite wash is so exclusive that it's not available in the cosmetic section. It dates back thousands of years, even to Cleopatra herself, who ruled just before Jesus was born. She was famous for her skin regimen of luxurious milk baths and wrote a "best-selling" book on beauty. Sadly, the book didn't survive, but her famed insistence on milk for her skin lives on. Like her, women in biblical times loved to wash their faces in milk, and often made this part of their morning routine.

BEAUTY SECRETS OF THE BIBLE (BSB) RICH MILK WASH

1   cup powdered goat's milk (try Meyenberg milk, listed in the Resource Guide)
1   cup quick-cooking oats

Process the powdered milk and oats in a blender or food processor until the mixture is very fine. Store in an airtight container, in a cool place, for up to four weeks.

To cleanse face, sprinkle a small amount of powder into the palm of your hand and mix into a paste with warm water. Massage onto face and rinse.

In the winter, when your skin is dry from indoor heating and the outside elements, try grinding fresh flaxseed into the oats as well. The essential fatty acids, called omega-3s, add extra emollients and are a rich addition to this wash.

Try this natural cleanser for one week and see the difference! This wash is good for most skin types and also a good choice for African-American women who often need extra help combating the build-up of dry skin, using gentle exfoliation and moisture. You can use the wash anywhere you want to pamper your skin.

The lactic acids in the milk are a natural source of alpha hydroxy acids that help fight the signs of aging, and the oats soothe and manually exfoliate the skin. Together, these ingredients will leave your skin unbelievably soft and supple.

> Milk is the first food for new life: Newborns are sustained by it, and the "land of milk and honey" was a reference to the cherished Promised Land, which represented the blessing of God's abundance and a new life for God's people. Peter even used milk to symbolize deep, nourishing truth, telling us we are to "desire the pure milk of the word" (I Pet. 2:2).

Although you can substitute other powdered milks in this recipe, goat's milk is my favorite because it feels so rich on the skin, is made by companies that do not use growth hormones, and is becoming increasingly chic. (Most powdered cow's milk is nonfat, which is not the best. We need those milk fats to make our skin feel wonderful.) Plus, goat's milk was more common in biblical days than cow's milk.

If you wear heavy makeup, you may need to remove the makeup first with a gentle commercial cleanser.

STEP TWO: NOURISH AND PLUMP

Christopher Watt is the facial care expert to the most famous faces in the world and has been featured in dozens of beauty publications. His work has led him to rediscover one of the most ancient products known to woman—honey. Christopher uses honey on his celebrity clients and graciously agreed to share his tips with us. Every woman I know balks at the idea of honey on the skin. We imagine it being sticky or syrupy. But since the most famous women in the world trust Christopher with their faces, I decided to take a chance with him as well.

HONEY TONIC
Apply 1–2 drops honey to wet fingertips and massage onto wet face. Do not rinse. Pat dry.

*H*oney was valuable in biblical days. Women applied it to their skin, along with oils, as part of their bathing ritual. Because of its value, it was part of the bribe offered to Joseph for the release of Benjamin back to his father, before Joseph's true identity was revealed (Gen. 43:11).

Honey is extolled throughout Scripture:

Honey is the promise of abundance in the Promised Land
(Ex. 3:17).

The judgments of the Lord are sweeter than honey (Psa. 19:10).

The Word of the Lord is sweeter than honey (Psa. 119:103).

The beloved bride's mouth is sweet like honey
(Song of Sol. 5:1).

The words we speak are like honey—sweet and nourishing
(Prov. 16:24).

"Honey is not sticky when used on damp skin," Christopher reassured me. "Honey works to give the skin a beautiful glow and to plump up fine lines. It's a natural humectant and exfoliant, and gives the skin better absorption of product."

Honey helps the skin attract and retain moisture, and helps absorb the moisturizer you apply after cleansing. Packed with nutrients and enzymes, honey helps counteract the pollution and harmful effects of the environment. Using honey as a routine step in your skin care regimen will help reduce fine lines and wrinkles, as well as aid in treating breakouts. Honey helps fight aging by helping the skin rebuild collagen and elastin, and according to Christopher, "nourishes, rejuvenates, and feeds the skin."

You simply have to try it to believe it. The first time I used the Honey Tonic, my husband walked into the bathroom as I was inspecting my skin, and remarked, "Your skin is glowing."

I also found that honey works well in treating razor burn. Because I have extremely fair, sensitive skin, I look like a chicken that's just been deplumed when I shave my legs. Every little hair follicle is red and irritated and stands out against my pale skin. I've tried many different remedies, but patting my damp legs down with a fine touch of honey soothes the inflammation and helps them absorb the moisturizer I use next.

BUYING HONEY

Buy raw honey because it has the most enzymes, Christopher says. Some honeys are pasteurized, which can destroy the enzymes. I find raw honey in the health food section of my favorite grocer.

Experiment with your favorite varieties—some are made from bees who feed on flowers, some are made from bees who feed on clover. While scientists are still working to unlock the differences between the honeys, they do know that the darker the honey, the richer it is in mineral content. All of the honeys, however, have key enzymes in common.

Honey's Sweet Little Secrets

*H*oney contains:

24 sugars
11–21 amino acids
18 sugar acids
11 minerals
5 enzymes
At least 4 different proteins[1]

STEP THREE: MOISTURIZE AND PROTECT

Your skin needs moisture. According to Dr. Julian Omidi, a cosmetic surgeon and dermatologist featured on E! Entertainment

Television, dryness is a leading cause of premature aging. I used to think moisturizer was for women with dry skin. I didn't understand that I was robbing my complexion every time I skipped this step.

In fact, when I asked Dr. Omidi for his top facial skin care tips, his first tip was, "Women should use an emollient after their shower." (Emollient is simply another name for moisturizer.) Dr. Omidi recommends moisturizing your face as soon as you get out of the shower so that precious moisture isn't lost from your skin when you step from the humid shower into a dry bathroom. This is the optimum time to replenish your skin. And here's an optimum moisturizer: olive oil. Packed with nutrients and antioxidants, olive oil nourishes the skin without blocking pores. It's been used since biblical times and represents the beauty of a people devoted to Him:

> The LORD *called you a thriving olive tree with fruit beautiful in form.* (Jer. 11:16 NIV)

According to Exodus 30, God even requested that olive oil be used as the base for a sacred anointing oil to be used in the tabernacle and its contents, including the famed ark of the covenant. Olive oil was a staple in biblical times of a woman's beauty regimen as well, used to keep the skin soft and supple.

OLIVE OIL MOISTURIZER
Place 2–3 drops of extra-virgin, organic olive oil onto your palm. Rub palms together and pat your face gently.

Of course, olive oil is available today at every grocer in America. Interestingly, as science has caught up with God in proving how nourishing olive oil can be for our bodies—both inside and out—cosmetics companies are cashing in. You can buy a one-ounce bottle of olive oil for $35 from a leading beauty company, and you can find olive oil in many pricey commercial products. But save your money: I can buy a bottle of premium organic olive oil at $10 for twelve ounces from my local grocery store and get incredible results. (As with any ingredient in this book, I do recommend buying organic. You'll find suggestions for places to buy in our Resource Guide. The extra-virgin varieties contain more antioxidant phytonutrients than the other varieties.)

"Won't my skin feel greasy?" is the most common question I hear when I recommend olive oil. You're not using enough to sauté yourself in, but rather, 2–3 drops at a time, patted gently onto the skin. You won't feel greasy, or smell like an entrée at an Italian restaurant. Your skin will be soft, radiant, and nourished. Like me, you may never go back to commercial moisturizers again.

---

*T*wo notable women of the Bible relied on oil's benefits to prepare them to woo a man: Esther and Ruth. While we aren't told in Scripture what kind of oil they used, olive oil is a likely candidate because of its availability in the region and its established cosmetic use.

Before a girl could take her turn with King Xerxes, she had to complete twelve months of beauty treatments that were ordered for the women. For six months she was treated with oil. . . . (Esther 2:12 NCV)

Ruth was instructed that to catch Boaz's attention she should:

"Therefore wash yourself and anoint yourself [with oil], put on your best garment and go down to the threshing floor. . . ." (Ruth 3:3)

And remember, just as your face needs moisture as soon as you step out of the shower, your hands need moisture after every wash as well. Hands are often neglected and can show a woman's age before her face. Place a small spritzer of olive oil next to your hand soap in the bathroom and kitchen, and nourish your skin every time you wash your hands. Your cuticles will benefit, too.

Using these exclusive, homemade products isn't just good for your skin: it's good for your wallet. I calculated the costs of following this regimen for one year versus one year of buying commercial products, and here are the savings:

Commercial exfoliating cleanser: $84 ($21 per 6-ounce bottle, 4 bottles a year)
BSB Rich Milk Wash: $48 (4 jars milk at $10 each, 2 boxes oats at $4 each)

Commercial fine lines plumper: $157 ($39.25 per half-ounce, 4 jars a year)
BSB Honey Tonic: $16 ($8 per 8-ounce jar, two jars per year)

Commercial olive oil moisturizer: $140 ($35 per ounce, 4 bottles per year)
BSB Olive Oil Moisturizer: $20 ($10 per 12 ounces, two bottles a year)

TOTAL SAVINGS: $297 per year!

FEED YOUR SKIN FROM THE INSIDE OUT

Premature aging can be accelerated when our skin isn't fed well from the inside, particularly when we're not eating enough antioxidant-rich foods, which protect us from skin-damaging free radicals. (Free radicals are simply molecules gone bad, attacking your cells to cause cell alteration or death. Free radicals are believed to be responsible for a certain degree of the visible signs of aging by attacking the skin's structure, including its collagen.) Fortunately, antioxidants play a major role in fighting free radicals, and the foods found in the Bible are some of the richest sources of antioxidants.

These natural foods that supply antioxidants are a great way to increase your energy, fight premature aging, protect yourself against cancer, keep your weight normal, and create gorgeous, glowing skin. (Who else but God can create foods that multitask like this?) Some of the healthiest foods mentioned in the Bible can also help keep your skin beautiful.

ALMONDS

In Chapter Two, we talked about the biblical symbolism of the almond, and how it reminds us to watch for God's faithful fulfillment of His promises to us. God also used the almond to perform a miracle among the Israelites: He caused the staff of Aaron, Moses' brother, to burst into blooms with ripe almonds (Num. 17:8). This staff was kept inside the ark of the covenant for remembrance. Scientists haven't been able to find the famed ark, but they have found some key facts about almonds. Almonds are a good source of vitamin E, a vitamin that is believed to protect against photodamage and wrinkles, and may even improve skin texture.[2]

APRICOTS

Did you know that apricots are believed to be the "forbidden fruit" of the Garden of Eden? Apple trees were not indigenous to the biblical lands, and the word *apple* is used in the Bible as a reference to the apricot. For example, Proverbs 25:11 compares a beautiful word to a beautiful apricot nestled in a silver serving dish: "A word fitly spoken is like apples of gold in settings of silver." Today, we know that apricots are rich sources of carotene, a phytonutrient that helps protect skin against harmful UV rays.[3]

PISTACHIOS

Pistachios were both eaten and used to make skin preparations in biblical times. They are believed to have been part of the Hanging Gardens of Babylon, built by the biblical king Nebuchadnezzar and considered to be one of the Seven Wonders of the Ancient World. Today, we know pistachios are rich in carotenoids, the phytonutrient that can help "block sunlight-induced inflammation of the skin, which leads to wrinkles."[4] As an added bonus, "one ounce of pistachios contains more fiber than a half-cup of spinach and the same amount as an orange or apple."[5] More fiber means you'll stay full longer, which helps with appetite control.

POMEGRANATES

Pomegranates were a luscious food in biblical times and are enjoying a resurgence in popularity today. During the Exodus, the Israelites complained loudly to Moses that he had led them into the wilderness and they didn't have pomegranates to eat. When Moses sent spies into the Promised Land, they brought back pomegranates. Pomegranates must be a favorite fruit of God's, too, because He commanded that their design be woven into the priest's robes and the architecture of the temple.

Today, this once-exotic fruit is available at most groceries every fall. Just split, drink the juice, and eat the seeds. When it's not available, buy 100 percent pure pomegranate juice, kept in the refrigerated section of the produce aisle.

Shown to contain more antioxidants than red wine or green tea, pomegranate juice is good for you inside and out.[6] Pomegranates are loaded with a particularly powerful type of antioxidant, called polyphenols, which fights aging and may also protect against heart disease. Many high-priced skin creams contain pomegranate extract to fight wrinkles, but it's always more fun to eat delicious fruits than apply a wrinkle cream.

WALNUTS

Although almonds and pistachios are the only nuts mentioned by name in the Bible, we know that walnuts were cultivated and enjoyed. In Mark 6, Jesus walks on water across the lake towards Gennesaret, a region that the ancient historian Josephus said was known for growing walnuts. Experts tell us that walnuts are a good source of omega-3 fatty acids, which are believed to help prevent dry skin and help the skin retain moisture. Consuming these essential fatty acids is also linked with a reduction in symptoms of psoriasis. Also, as discussed in Chapter Two, omega-3s have an anti-inflammatory effect. Many studies are being done to examine the role between inflammation and aging and you can expect to hear more about the overall benefits of consuming walnuts.

RAISINS

In Jeremiah 2:21, God calls Israel a "noble vine." The fruit of the vine—grapes and raisins—was much loved as food and drink. In 1 Samuel 25, a very wise, and very beautiful, woman named Abigail, took one hundred clusters of raisins, along with other foods, as a peace offering to David to persuade him to call off a deadly attack on her household. It worked. The Bible references raisins many times, usually as "cakes," which were simply dried raisins pressed together. Modern women know that raisins are antioxidant powerhouses. (Only the humble prune has more antioxidants than raisins.) And since a new study reports that people who eat antioxidant-rich foods will have fewer wrinkles, it's smart to add raisins into your daily snack routine.[7] I've included a recipe to get you started:

BSB TRAIL MIX

Mix equal parts of the following:
Raisins
Dried figs
Raw, whole almonds
Raw walnuts
Darkest chocolate chips

Set out in an attractive bowl and watch it disappear. This snack has synergy! It fights premature aging, excess weight, heart disease, and hunger pangs. (If you are a chronic breakfast-skipper, package this mix, minus the chocolate chips, into individual baggies and keep in the pantry or car. A healthy breakfast— instead of starving— helps return you to your natural weight.)

Dark Chocolate Chips

Okay, so these aren't mentioned in the Bible, but there is a fun connection between chocolate and God: nuns were the first to discover that it was delicious to mix cocoa with sugar.[8]

HELP FOR COMMON SKIN COMPLAINTS

Every woman battles skin woes at some point in her life. It's not uncommon to experience breakouts at the same time you're also noticing fine lines and wrinkles. If you need help battling a particular issue, the first step is to visit a dermatologist. This may come as a surprise in a book that focuses on natural healing and heavenly treatments, but I interviewed two of the country's top dermatologists for this book, and I was impressed with how modern medicine is returning to more natural approaches in skin care. Don't be shy about mixing "medicine and miracles." Healing and restoration are very often found through skilled practitioners who understand the balance between nature and science.

ACNE

Because acne can occur for a variety of reasons, an accurate diagnosis must come before a successful treatment. Many times, acne in women is related to monthly hormonal changes, and a doctor can assess what steps might be helpful in managing those lovely swings we all deal with. Other times, acne can be confused with other skin conditions.

Skin is designed to allow our pores to get rid of oil and skin cells every day. Sometimes this natural process becomes inhibited and a pore is blocked. Bacteria festers, and a pimple is born. (It's not unusual to have bacteria on and in our skin—our body houses 40 trillion bacteria!) So for skin to work properly, it's first important to avoid using products that prevent the pores from breathing—and remember that petroleum-based products may be a culprit.

But if isolated blemishes do appear, honey can come to your rescue again. Celebrities in particular can suffer from breakouts because of the heavy makeup they wear and the hot lights they work under, so Christopher Watt recommends a dab of honey on an impending pimple to help clear it up. (I loved this tip, as it dried up the pimple without drying my skin and without any flaking.)

There is mounting evidence that a healthy lifestyle like the one we're discussing in this book can help stabilize our hormonal swings and stress, which all contribute to breakouts. In particular, a healthy lifestyle can also prevent high blood sugar, which triggers the oil glands to produce more oil.

WRINKLES

Aging isn't a disease we need to cure. Most of have heard the admonition in Proverbs 31 that physical beauty quickly disap-

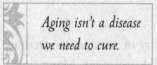
Aging isn't a disease we need to cure.

pears. But 1 Corinthians 13:13 (NIV) offers an interesting thought: "And now these three remain: faith, hope and love." Our bodies' strength will falter, lines will appear on our faces, and our breasts will fall down and not get up. But three things will remain with us and refuse to budge: faith, hope, and love, the very essence of profound beauty.

Fear of aging is only for those who believe in an absolute end of life; but for us, hope should permeate even our uneasiness about aging. Other women should see a visible difference in our attitude about aging: Women should see our *gratitude.* Life is fragile and fleeting. Gratitude for each new dawn softens our irritation over aging. We don't have to rejoice over wrinkles, but a gratitude for life—and most importantly, the expectation of a new life yet to come—can soften the lines we get from worry and grief over losing our youth.

It's important to know, however, that the natural aging process can be *artificially* accelerated by poor choices, so we can address those here. In particular, premature aging is accelerated by

Smoking
Obesity
Poor diet

Sun exposure
Stress
Poor skin care

There are proactive steps you can take to reduce or eliminate every artificial accelerant. Stop smoking, improve your diet to incorporate the foods we've discussed, and improve your skin care regimen. Two points, however, bear special mention: sun exposure and stress.

When I asked for the top tips for preventing premature aging, Dr. Omidi said, "Wear sunscreen. Most women think they can see sun damage. They think sun damage happens when you get burned and your skin is red. In reality, sun damage is happening even when they can't see it. You need to wear sunscreen every day, even on overcast days." I keep sunscreen everywhere: upstairs, downstairs, and even in my car. I use makeup with a built-in sunscreen, and apply sunscreen on top of this, remembering to also protect the other areas so prone to sun damage: hands, arms, and neck.

Stress is the other artificial accelerant. First, it disrupts our sleep, which inhibits our body's nightly repair work. Next, stress affects circulation to the skin: capillaries shrink, and blood flow to the skin decreases as the body redirects blood to the internal organs.[9] Stress naturally deepens the wrinkles we get when we make those unhappy, irritated faces. We don't call them "frown lines" for nothing.

Stress is best handled through what the Bible calls "a renewing of your mind." If ever there was a logical connection between spirit and beauty, this is it. Again, there is a synergy in God's creation and commands that applies here. We are encouraged throughout Scripture to spend quiet time in God's presence, praying and meditating, and to spend time with believers who will encourage us in our spiritual walk. Modern studies continue to confirm what God told us ages ago: prayer, reflection, and nurturing fellowship improve the quality of our lives and help to insulate us from stress.[10]

Exercise has also been proven a very effective stress reliever in many respected studies.[11] It fights cholesterol, heart disease, stress, obesity, mood swings, hormonal side effects from PMS and menopause, as well as protecting against cancer, boosting the immune system and the libido, and aiding in better sleep.

Finally, obesity is a surprising cause of overall premature aging. A study has correlated obesity to an extra 8.8 years of aging.[12] Achieving a natural weight is the result of making more natural choices, and you're moving in the right direction as you consider the suggestions in this book.

Aging isn't a disease, but *premature* aging is related to the processes of stress and disease, and it is worth fighting.

DRY SKIN

Combating dry skin can begin with removing harsh products from our bath routine, using gentler washes such as the Rich Milk Wash, and adding healthy foods into our diet that are rich in essential fatty acids, such as the almonds, flax, and fish that we discussed earlier. You may also wish to add a supplement of these oils into your diet as well, especially if dry skin is a problem for you. Try adding supplements of fish oil, flaxseed oil, black currant oil, or evening primrose oil. You can expect to wait six to eight weeks before you see results, but these oils are good for your whole body, not just your skin, so be patient and give them time to work. (See the Resource Guide for suggestions on supplement manufacturers.)

ECZEMA

My daughter suffers from eczema, and we've tried many different creams and lotions to soothe her skin, but nothing has worked as well for us as olive oil. Our pediatrician encouraged us to continue using the olive oil and warned us to stay away from baby oil and petroleum-based products, which, he says, tend to dry out the skin and make eczema worse. I certainly had no trouble following his advice when it was reported that the FDA chose to place a "black box" warning on two prescription eczema treatments because of a risk of cancer associated with their use.

A recent study showed that a homemade mixture of equal parts olive oil with unprocessed honey and beeswax is incredibly beneficial when applied topically to either eczema or psoriasis.[13] (You can check my website at www.gingergarrett.com for directions on mixing this.) Whenever you can use a natural treatment that gives good results, you can lessen your need for commercial products that may have unwanted side effects. Olive oil's healing properties for our skin are only beginning to be understood.

But don't just use olive oil on your skin—eat it, too! A new study reveals that the micronutrients in olive oil may improve circulation.[14] Doctors are excited about this find because it means that olive oil, rich in antioxidants, may protect the heart and fight heart disease by improving blood vessel function. This is not just good news for our hearts, but for our skin as well. There are a lot of beauty creams, gadgets, and lotions that promise to boost circulation to the skin and therefore enhance its vitality, but olive oil is an inexpensive, safe, and potentially powerful way to achieve the same goal—while improving your overall health as well.

When choosing an olive oil for beauty or for cooking, search for organic oils that are labeled "extra virgin." These have the highest amount of the micronutrient called phenols.

BEAUTY BONUSES

What woman hasn't envied Queen Esther, who spent a year being pampered from head to toe with beauty treatments as she readied herself to meet the King of Persia? Today's woman has a hard time finding ten minutes for extra beauty treats! So below, I am going to give you a few fast, fabulous treats with wonderful connections to our spiritual heritage.

MUD MASKS

Mud masks are great to do before a special evening out or on a lazy weekend morning before you jump in the shower. (Don't make *my* mistake of applying a mud mask when expecting a UPS delivery, or all your future packages will be thrown out from the truck at high speed.)

Try masks made with mud from the Dead Sea, also called the Salt Sea in the Bible. The "Dead" Sea is named such because there's no aquatic life there: it has the highest salinity of any body of water in the world, slightly over 30 percent, with a rich concentration of minerals such as calcium, potassium, bromide, and magnesium. In the Bible the Dead Sea is mentioned several times, once in connection with a miracle. In Joshua 3, waters flowing into the Dead Sea were stopped so that the Israelites could cross the Jordan River safely. The waters stopped at the moment the priests carrying the ark of the covenant stepped into the water. The Dead Sea also marked the border for the tribe of Judah in the Promised Land.

With the richest mineral content of any body of water, scientists have studied the mud of the Dead Sea for many dermatological conditions. Dead Sea mud has shown to be a promising treatment for psoriasis and dermatitis.

Dead Sea mud is also famous as a cosmetic treatment, particularly in mud masks for the face. In my own experiments with Dead

Sea masks versus other clay and mineral masks, I have noticed a substantial difference. The masks that are made exclusively of Dead Sea mud tend to absorb oil without drying or irritating the skin. Other clay masks will produce a stronger flush from irritation.

As with any cosmetic product, you'll want to read the label. Some products claim to be Dead Sea mud, but in reality contain very little of the precious mud.

BATH TREATS

Have you ever noticed how profoundly refreshed you feel after a soak in the tub? Bathing is not only refreshing, but good for us too. It's a fantastic way to relieve stress, contemplate the day, and meditate on God's goodness. Adding scent sweetens the experience. A study reported in the *International Journal of Cosmetic Science* found that women who took scented baths were more relaxed than women who took unscented baths.[15]

You can add ingredients such as the following to the water and treat your skin to added benefits, while you soothe stress and combat premature aging.

BSB Rich Milk Cleanser for dry, irritated skin. Try this after a day at the beach, or when exposed to the elements. It's especially wonderful on winter nights, so your skin feels soft and supple all night. Itchy, dry skin can wreck a good night's sleep.

Bath salts for sore muscles. Mineral baths, including Dead Sea salts, are shown to help alleviate skin conditions such as psoriasis and help the body renew tired muscles.

Rosemary. A principal scent in many expensive bath products, fresh rosemary is an antioxidant with a scent that deeply revitalizes you. Gather a group of stems, tie with a ribbon, tie the ribbon to the faucet, and allow water to pour over as the tub fills. There is a wonderful legend about rosemary: the legend says that when Mary and Joseph were fleeing to protect the infant Jesus from the wicked king Herod, they stopped to rest for the night. Mary draped her robe over a nearby bush, and it burst into bloom overnight, taking on the color and fragrance of her robe. It is known forever more as the rose of Mary, or rosemary.

Lavender. Another easy-to-grow herb that is unbelievably delicious to smell is lavender. A few sprigs at the bedside and a few sprigs into the tub water are an indulgent way to soothe stress. If you don't have fresh lavender, you can buy dried lavender in bulk anywhere soap supplies are sold. Put a handful into some cheesecloth or sheer fabric, and tie under faucet as above.

The ancient Greek name for lavender was *nard,* and biblical translations vary between using the words *nard* and *spikenard.* Because of the similarities of the names, some believe that lavender may be referenced in some stories as the famed nard of the Bible, a perfume costly and indulgent.

Rose petals. Don't throw out that flower because it has started to wilt! Shake a rose that has wilted slightly into the tub and enjoy the beauty and fragrance of the petals. Long the symbol of complete and eternal love, they make a perfect backdrop for our bath. Roses are mentioned in Scripture, but we can't assume this "rose" is the same flower as our modern red rose. Many plants we can find at the local nursery with biblical names such as "rose of Jericho" or "rose of Sharon" are the result of medieval monks who loved the biblical stories as much as we do, and created gardens that honored these stories. Since the monks possessed no firsthand knowledge of biblical flora, they identified local plants that seemed appropriate or resembled some biblical person, object, or motif, and linked it explicitly with the Bible by name. Many of these identifications have remained and become part of plant lore.[16]

*F*ix yourself a tray of goodies to enjoy while in the tub to get the maximum benefit to your spirit, mind, and body. Have cold, fresh berries or a beautiful, for-bath-time-only goblet filled with chilled pomegranate juice close at hand, or have instrumental music or hymns playing while you relax.

FRANKINCENSE AND MYRRH

No other biblical oils are as famous, perhaps, as frankincense and myrrh. The gift of the Wise Men to the infant Jesus, these two precious oils have been used throughout history to soften the skin and prevent wrinkles, and as holy perfumes. Esther was covered in oil of myrrh for six months to perfect her skin: "Before a girl's turn came to go in to King Xerxes, she had to complete twelve months of beauty treatments prescribed for the women, six months with oil of myrrh . . ." (Esther 2:12 NIV).

Myrrh and frankincense are still available today. The unusual aroma of each is rich, spicy, and woodsy, and transports us to biblical days and beloved figures from Scripture.

I buy essential oils of myrrh and frankincense at my local Whole Foods Market®. (Essential oils are simply highly concentrated versions of natural oils extracted from plants and plant matter such as fruit, bark, and leaves. Because the oils are concentrated, one tiny bottle will last for a very long time.) I use them to create these beauty treats that you'll want to try. It's important to buy these oils at a store where you can test the scent before you buy. Inferior oils of frankincense and myrrh will have a bad "paint thinner" odor. High quality oils will smell rich and warm.

MYRRH FACIAL SPRITZ

In a small spritzer bottle, combine purified water with 1–2 drops of myrrh essential oil. (Each manufacturer will give more specific diluting ratios on the bottle for their brand of oil.) I use this spritz to set my makeup, refresh my skin throughout the day, replenish moisture, and also for a fast stress-relieving break.

FRANKINCENSE AND MYRRH BATH SALTS: THE WISE (WO)MAN'S GIFTS

Make a batch of these and nestle the package in a gold basket for a beautiful presentation that mimics the Wise Men's gifts of frankincense, gold, and myrrh. These make great bathtime luxuries for yourself and wonderful holiday gifts. What a sweet way to share the message of Christmas. The recipe below makes enough for ten baths.

6   cups sea salt (Dead Sea salt is preferable; or use coarse sea salt)
3   cups Epsom salt
1   cup baking soda

Combine the sea salt, Epsom salt, and baking soda. Add 5 drops each of frankincense and myrrh essential oil, or until the mixture is richly scented. (You can also add in a sweet scent like lavender or orange to soften the smoky, spicy tones.)

Combine well and scoop one cup each into ten containers.

(You can use cellophane baggies, colored plastic wrap tied with ribbon, ceramic jars—use your imagination!) Nestle the salts inside a gold basket with a Christmas card from you.

Frankincense, valued for thousands of years as a liniment, perfume and biblical gift, may have a new use: cancer treatment.
—FOX NEWS[17]

*F*rankincense made international news when it was revealed that it has shown promise as a treatment for malignant melanomas in early animal studies. Horses with these cancers were treated with both topical and injected frankincense and all showed improvement. Scientists are working to uncover frankincense's secrets and understand how we can take advantage of its potential in humans suffering from skin cancer.

5

Beauty Secrets: Hair

Hair has been a source of fascination and romantic attraction throughout the ages. Our ancient sisters spent hours arranging and setting their hair, using elaborate combs and pins to perfect the designs. All wore long hair and many set it in curls. Even Solomon, the wisest man to ever live, was held captive by the fascination of his beloved's hair: "Your hair is like royal tapestry; the king is held captive by its tresses. How beautiful you are and how pleasing, O love, with your delights!" (Song of Sol. 7:5–6 NIV)

God pays special attention to our hair as well. Did you know that it is a symbol of His loving protection and provision? Listen as He compares our value to a little bird:

> Are not two sparrows sold for a copper coin? And not one of them falls to the ground apart from your Father's will. But the very hairs of your head are all numbered. Do not fear therefore; you are of more value than many sparrows. (Matt. 10:29–31)

Has anyone ever been so in love with you that he would attempt to count every hair on your head? Who has ever watched vigilantly over you in your sleep, in your work, noticing the most minute detail such as one fallen hair? Your hair is a constant reminder that God is involved in every daily detail of your life. Nothing about you escapes His attention.

How to Choose a Shampoo

My basic rule for choosing a good shampoo is this: you should understand the label when you read it. Look for a list of ingredients you know and recognize, such as almond oil and rosemary extract. Because these "all natural" shampoos usually don't contain harsh ingredients like sodium laurel sulfate, they probably won't irritate your scalp and leave it itchy like some commercial shampoos.

COMMON HAIR CONCERNS AND CURES

If your tresses are suffering from distresses, there are some wonderful—and wonderfully simple—remedies to restore the natural luster and good health of your hair. Dandruff, dry hair, and the frizzies all are problems that can be tamed with a few smart solutions.

DANDRUFF

If you fear wearing black because of unsightly flakes, you may be surprised to hear what causes dandruff. Although most people assume dandruff comes from a dry scalp, the opposite is true: people with oily scalps tend to suffer most from dandruff.[1]

What natural remedies are available that can combat dandruff?

1. Lower your stress level. Stress has been linked with rising levels of androgen, a hormone produced by the adrenal glands. Androgen has a link to dandruff because it is believed to increase scalp oil, and therefore increase dandruff flakes. By reducing stressors and incorporating prayer and reflection into your life, you can take a positive step toward eliminating dandruff naturally.

2. Eat more biblical foods for essential fatty acids. Many experts recommend adding flaxseed to your diet to treat dandruff from the "inside out." Because flaxseed is high in essential fatty acids (EFAs) that help promote healthy skin, adding flaxseed to your diet can improve the condition of your scalp. Remember, many of the biblical foods we've talked about are high in EFAs. You can also supplement your diet with flax oil, fish oil, or black currant oil as you change your diet.

Another addition to your diet to help combat dandruff (as well as acne) is zinc, a mineral that is found in almonds and beans.

3. Use vinegar as a topical treatment. In addition to making sure you get enough essential fatty acids, try using vinegar as a topical treatment to kill another suspected cause of dandruff. The alpha hydroxy acids in apple cider vinegar kill the fungus and bacteria that may help cause dandruff.[2] A spritz bottle in the shower can be used to apply it directly to the scalp. Vinegar is as old as the Bible itself and part of the common culture. Different flavored vinegars were made and sold in biblical times, and vinegar was commonplace in cooking and preserving foods. For beauty treatments, I use organic apple cider vinegar with "mother" in it. It's inexpensive, and contains healthy enzymes that are destroyed during the commercial bottling process other manufacturers use. You may see a little cloud floating in it—that's called the "mother," a naturally occurring part of the process that converts alcohol into acetic acid, the key ingredient in vinegar.

Do Babies Get Dandruff, Too?

One of the more common frustrations of a new mom is seeing her beautiful baby develop ugly yellow clumps of oily, patchy skin on the scalp. It looks like giant flakes of dandruff, but there is a simple, safe way to treat it, according to the FDA: The scaly scalp inflammation is common in newborn babies, although it can occur anytime in infancy. Rubbing warm olive oil . . . into the baby's scalp and leaving it on overnight can loosen and soften scales, which can be washed off the next day with a mild shampoo.[3]

DULL HAIR

Rosemary's fragrance is found in many high-end hair care products because of its rejuvenating scent and its purported ability to stimulate hair growth and relieve itchy scalps. Rosemary is also said to give your hair a lovely sheen.

Rosemary is one of the easiest herbs to grow. I keep two rosemary bushes in containers on my porch. They are evergreen, low maintenance, hard to kill, and when my guests brush past them to enter my home, they release a lovely scent. I can also clip a few fresh leaves whenever I am cooking, or when I need an extra bit of shine in my hair on a special occasion.

To use rosemary to give your hair extra shine, boil several stems of rosemary in natural spring water (if available) and use the cooled water as a final rinse. After using rosemary, I find that I can skip conditioner, which is an added benefit since my hair is fine and easily weighed down.

Another option, and a faster one, is to use rosemary essential oil in a deep conditioning hair masque, which we'll reveal later in the chapter.

DRY HAIR AND FLY-AWAYS

Once again, olive oil comes to our rescue, replenishing hair in several ways:

- ❖ Use a few drops of olive oil as a light conditioner in the shower by rubbing it between your palms and running your hands through your hair before rinsing.
- ❖ For deep conditioning, use a more generous amount of olive oil and wrap hair in a warm towel. (To quickly warm a towel, pop one in the dryer on high for a few minutes.) Leave oil treatment on for at least 10 minutes before shampooing out.
- ❖ Two to three drops of olive oil rubbed between your palms can be used to smooth out fly-away hairs and frizzies.

HAIR LOSS

If you're experiencing hair loss, the first step is to get a check-up with your doctor. Hair loss can signal underlying disorders, especially with your thyroid. After your doctor has given you a thumbs up on your health, you can investigate some natural remedies.

While there are many commercial products that claim to restore a healthy hairline, examining your diet is a smart first step. There are several biblical foods that may help boost your body's ability to nourish hair. First is the B vitamin biotin, a vitamin found in almonds. In a study of patients who were severely diet-deficient in biotin and experiencing hair loss, the *American Journal of Clinical Nutrition* found that "Supplementation . . . 200 micrograms biotin per day resulted in gradual regrowth of healthy hair."[4]

Biotin works by helping our bodies produce keratin. Keratin is a protein that nourishes our skin and nails. If your diet is poor, and you are not consuming healthy amounts of biotin, your hair and nails may suffer. Biotin is produced in our bodies and is in many natural foods, but we can become deficient in it in several ways. A study found that "while deficiency in biotin is somewhat rare, it sometimes occurs in individuals taking a long-term regimen of antibiotics, or those on a calorie-restricted diet for a considerable length of time."[5]

So if you incorporate almonds into your diet, you may help prevent hair loss. And you can ask your doctor about adding in additional biotin supplements as needed.

Adding foods high in essential fatty acids can also help. Flaxseed in particular adds a powerful punch of lignans, fiber, and fatty acids and has a rich, nutty taste. Best of all, adding it into your diet can be as simple as taking a supplement or sprinkling a bit on your cereal or yogurt: "Adding two tablespoons of ground flaxseed to your daily diet . . . will slow down the fallout by helping to balance the high levels of hormones behind hair loss."[6]

Flaxseed is best when fresh. Buy a coffee grinder and use it for flaxseeds—keep it near your cereal bowls for a gentle daily reminder. I urge you to consider using fresh flax over the supplements, because freshly ground flaxseeds contain a healthy dose of fiber.

DAMAGED HAIR

A study was conducted to compare three of the hair care industry's more popular oils. Which oil would protect the hair from protein damage? Which oil would be able to penetrate the hair shaft more effectively? The conclusion: coconut oil. Among three oils, coconut oil was the only oil found to reduce the protein loss remarkably for both undamaged and damaged hair when used as a pre-wash and post-wash grooming product.[7]

African-American women can especially benefit from coconut oil's ability to help "heal" damaged hair. Women of color complain frequently that certain products, especially relaxers, damage their hair. But coconut oil is an easy remedy to try, and best of all, it's inexpensive and a great body moisturizer, too. In the later biblical days, coconuts were a luxury item, available only to the powerful and wealthy. Think of it as the "plasma TV" of the biblical world. Today, you can find it in the health foods section at your local grocer.

Keep a jar of coconut oil in the bathroom and use it to precondition your hair by rubbing through the damaged ends before shampooing, or for a special treat, use our deep conditioning and shine masque recipe found below. Because coconut oil so thoroughly penetrates the hair, you may need to shampoo twice afterwards. Use the gentlest shampoo you can find (skip the sodium laurel sulfate we mentioned earlier), and be prepared to fall in love with your hair.

BSB DEEP SHINE AND REPAIR HAIR MASQUE

¼ cup coconut oil

2 drops rosemary essential oil or 2 drops lavender essential oil

Combine and store in refrigerator. Use 2–4 tablespoons per treatment. Work into damp hair and cover with a warm towel, fresh from the dryer. Let set for ten minutes before shampooing.

This masque is especially wonderful after a day at the

beach or pool, when your hair feels coarse and dry from the surf and chlorine.

Cost per year:

Commercial repair masque: $140 per year ($35 per 4-ounce treatment, 4 jars per year)

BSB Deep Shine and Repair Hair Masque: $20 per year ($10 for one 14-ounce jar coconut oil, $10 for one bottle essential oil)

TOTAL SAVINGS: $120 per year

GRAY HAIR

What woman isn't a little annoyed to find a few gray hairs sneaking up on her? After all, most of us feel like we're not really aging—we're simply teenagers with a lot of life experience! Going gray isn't only about accepting our age; it's about changing our identity. We identify ourselves with and by our hair color: the blondes have more fun, the dark-haired girls are so mysterious and smart, and the redheads have fiery natures. But women with beautiful white hair, or silvery shimmers of gray, give us a different glimpse of beauty that is powerfully affirming. The Bible, too, offers some affirming words on gray hair:

> *Gray hair is a mark of distinction. . . .* (Prov. 16:31 MSG)

> *Gray hair is a crown of splendor. . . .* (Prov. 16:31 NIV)

That's a beautiful sentiment, and a good note to end this chapter on. May we all live well and long to achieve a crown of splendor.

✑ 6 ✑

Beauty Secrets: Cosmetics

In biblical times, women loved cosmetics as much as we do today. They painted their eyes, lips, cheeks, and powdered their faces. They even invented glitter eye shadow, made by drying and crushing glittery beetle wings. (Isn't it comforting to think of a mother living three thousand years ago, shouting at her daughter, "You're not going out of this tent with that eye shadow on!")

The basis for ancient makeup was minerals. They used the minerals easily available to them, especially galena, ochre, stibnite, and malachite. Mixing these minerals with olive oil or animal fat, they painted them on, much as we use an eye shadow brush to apply our own makeup.

Today, minerals as makeup have made an incredible comeback. Women are looking for natural alternatives in every aspect of their beauty routine.

There are dozens of mineral-based makeup lines to choose from, and I've listed quite a few in the Resource Guide. When shopping for a mineral makeup, always read the label. Many inexpensive "mineral" powders I've found at mass retailers are actually a blend of minerals and synthetics. Look for mineral makeups that are free from synthetic colors, fragrances, and preservatives.

MINERAL MAKEUP

Mineral-based cosmetics have made a phenomenal comeback in recent years, first embraced by dermatologists and plastic surgeons who needed gentle, nonirritating cosmetics for patients. The cosmetic industry latched on to the idea and the minerals revolution was born. Because we're a global economy, cosmetic companies weren't limited to the natural resources on hand: they could choose their minerals based on our needs. You'll find most mineral makeups are formulated from zinc oxide, titanium dioxide, and mica. (If zinc oxide sounds familiar to you, it's because it is used as a sunscreen.) Minerals offer distinct advantages over other types of makeup:

+ They have built-in protection from UVA and UVB rays (check the label for exact SPF).
+ They are nonirritating.
+ They won't clog pores.
+ Their rich pigments last longer.

Michelle Doan, founder and artistic director of Emani Professional Cosmetics, shared her expertise with us. Michelle reminded me that a lot of makeups aren't good for the skin, and are made from cheap ingredients. "Talc is an inexpensive filler used in a lot of makeup. I can buy talc for $1 per kilo, while some minerals cost as much as $300 per kilo." Talc, while inexpensive, causes the color to dissipate, and you need to apply it frequently to freshen the color.

Pure mineral makeup is richly pigmented. Mineral makeup, Michelle explains, is 98 percent pigment, while mass makeup brands can be 98 percent talc. With such richly pigmented colors, a little goes a long way and they give a beautiful finish that synthetics can't imitate. As an experiment, I applied two identical shades of gold eye shadow on my wrist. One was synthetic, and one was made of pure minerals. I asked my husband if he could tell a difference. He picked the mineral one immediately as looking the most natural. There was a sheen to it that made it glow, versus the chunky, fake sparkle of the synthetic version.

True mineral makeup also boasts other advantages over synthetics:

- ✤ Minerals catch and diffuse light, giving your face a radiant glow and softening the appearance of flaws and wrinkles.
- ✤ Minerals look more natural than synthetic colors.
- ✤ And, Michelle tells us, "Minerals provide a barrier to protecting the skin from free radicals and the environment." She also points out the irony that the companies selling us synthetic makeup that can irritate, clog, and dull our complexions are the same companies selling us rejuvenating treatments and creams.

Mineral makeup is good for your skin, but is it good for your wallet? Those little jars of powder can seem expensive for what you're getting. We're conditioned to judging the value of makeup by its size and cost. When you remember that mass makeup products can be loaded with cheap fillers, and that mineral makeup is pigment-packed, you can begin to see the real test of a makeup. A tiny sprinkle of mineral makeup goes a long way. The eye colors, in particular, amaze me for how very little I need to get a good result, and how long the container lasts. They also last longer throughout the day, which means I don't have to reapply.

As with any cosmetic, you may want to sample a few mineral powders to find the one that best suits you. Some have more of a shimmer to them than others, and some require a two-step process of foundation and setting powder to achieve a finished look. Many times you can purchase sample sizes online, or try the lines in retail stores. (See the Resource Guide for more information.) Jane Iredale, founder of Jane Iredale Mineral Cosmetics, advises women to "try one brand on one side of the face and another brand on the other. If the makeup doesn't last all day without minimum touch-ups, isn't water resistant and doesn't feel weightless on the skin, then . . . look for another line."

EYES AND LIPS

Like ancient women, most of our efforts to apply cosmetics focus on our eyes and lips. Ancient women wanted to visually enlarge their eyes, and they often stained their lips red as well. Lips and eyes are a focal point of every woman's beauty routine.

With our eyes we see the world, but only God can give us proper perspective of the events that shape our life:

God can open our eyes and help us see situations clearly
(Gen. 21:19; 2 Kings 6:19–21).

With our eyes we witness the miracles of God, and we should remember them forever (Deut. 1:29–31; Deut. 4:8–10).

God remembers every tear that falls from our eyes, and someday, God will wipe away every tear from our eyes (Ps. 56:7–9; Rev. 7:16–17).

In researching everything the Scriptures say about both, it became clear that eyes and lips also shape our lives in unexpected ways. We spend time every day drawing attention to each—and so has every other generation of women, right back through the ages to our biblical sisters. With our eyes we take in creation and witness the memories that will replay in our minds for the rest of our lives. With our lips, we speak the words that will nurture or destroy. It is fitting, therefore, that these receive special attention in both our physical and spiritual lives.

King Solomon, one of the more prolific writers in the Bible, had quite a lot to say about our lips and mouths. In a letter to his son, the book of Proverbs, he told us that the mouth of the righteous is a "well of life," and "wisdom is found on the lips" (Prov. 10:11, 13).

Solomon also wrote a book about his love affair with his bride and described her beautiful lips: "Your lips are like a strand of scarlet, and your mouth is lovely. . . . Your lips, O my spouse, drip as the honeycomb" (Song of Sol. 4:3, 11).

Solomon understood that our mouths and lips are more than just the object of romantic fascination; they can bless the world with wisdom and life-affirming words.

USING ALOE VERA TO PREP YOUR EYES AND LIPS

Aloe vera is renowned for its ability to help skin heal. It's loaded with active compounds, and has been shown to increase collagen production.[1] Aloe vera has been studied in major hospitals and has been a part of alternative medicine for generations. It is a hardy plant that will endure neglect, thrives despite a minimal amount of care, and provides good results.

But aloe is a tricky plant to process commercially. The inner rind of the leaf contains a powerful laxative. You can't simply grind up an aloe plant and throw it in your juice without rather dramatic results. Aloe juice must be expressed, leaving the inner rind intact. Thankfully, it's easy to do this by hand at home. Simply snip off the end of the leaf, and squeeze. The precious gel will come right out.

This aloe gel is made of powerful active compounds and nutrients that include vitamins, amino acids, and minerals. Studies are still being done to understand the components of aloe and how they all work together, but one of the primary reasons it is believed to assist topical healing is because of its ability to attract and hold moisture. (When shopping for aloe vera plants, look for the common species labeled as *Aloe barbadensis*. It's the one most often studied by medical researchers and skin experts.)

The humble aloe vera plant is mentioned several times in Scripture:

God's robes are said to be perfumed with aloe, myrrh, and cassia: "All thy garments smell of myrrh, and aloes, and cassia . . ." (Ps. 45:8 KJV).

The homes of God's people spreading out are wonderful to see, "like aloes planted by the LORD" (Num. 24:5–7).

Moisture is exactly what we need around our lips and those fine lines around our eyes, and aloe's active, healing compounds may bind moisture and help "plump" the skin.

So every morning before I apply lipstick, I cut a tiny end off of my aloe vera plant. I squeeze out the juice and pat it onto my lips and into the fine lines around my mouth that are beginning to develop. It takes a brief moment to dry, then I apply my liner and lipstick as usual. The aloe vera juice makes a fabulous base for lip products, and my lips do indeed look fuller, because the lipstick gets a better application and my lips stay moisturized. Try it—you'll be amazed at how well the aloe vera clings to your lips. Use it in place of your lip plumper, and use it to make any lipstick a long-lasting one. I also use any extra aloe gel to dip my makeup brush into before applying my powdered mineral shadows. It replaces more expensive "eye shadow foundation creams."

We all love full lips. Over-the-counter lip plumpers work on the principle that if you irritate the skin and cause increased blood to flow to the area, your lips will puff up. I just don't think a healthy long-term beauty plan should involve irritating the skin several times a day. They also contain questionable ingredients, including collagen, which is often manufactured from slaughterhouse waste.

But there is a better solution: aloe vera.

Lip plumper: $40

Cost of aloe vera plant: $3

TOTAL SAVINGS: $148 per year (based on buying 4 lip plumping products per year, versus 4 plants per year)

You can also use the gel as a "base" for your foundation. Simply pat any excess gel onto your face before applying foundation. It soothes irritated skin and will give your skin the feeling of an expensive lifting and firming cream.

SETTING YOUR MAKEUP

To set your makeup, and to be refreshed throughout the day, I make facial spritzers to keep handy. I keep one in my desk, one in the bathroom, and one in the fridge. My favorites are lavender, rosewater, myrrh, and green tea. Organic lavender water and rosewater are easy to find at any natural foods store, so I simply pour those into small spritzers and I'm done. I've shared the recipe for myrrh facial spritz on page 94. For the green tea spritzer, whenever I brew tea to drink, I pour the cooled leftover tea into a bottle. It's that simple.

These are all incredibly refreshing spritzers that reduce stress while refreshing your skin. The delicate scents encourage you to slow down and take a deep breath, and they refresh your skin.

HIGHLIGHTING CHEEKBONES

After you've applied and set your makeup, there's one last trick you can try to highlight your cheekbones. Put two to three drops of olive oil in your palms and rub together. With the heel of your hand, press against the upper ridge of each cheekbone, under the eye and back toward your hairline.

The effect is subtle and stunning. It creates a glow to your appearance without makeup. It looks natural and yet the eye is drawn to "see" cheekbones. This is a great tip for daytime, when you may not want to use shimmer powders to highlight the cheekbones, but still want to have a healthy glow.

MORNING COSMETIC ROUTINE

1. After following the BSB Three-Step Skin Regimen (see pages 73–80), gently pat concealer under eyes where needed.

2. Sweep mineral foundation across face, sweeping in circular, downward motions. (If you sweep upward, you'll make your tiny facial hairs stand up and out.)

3. Apply aloe vera to lips and use any excess to wet eye shadow brush.

4. Apply mineral eye shadow. A light color should sweep across entire eyelid all the way to the eyebrows, including a little dot of light color at the inner corner of eyes. A darker color should go just above the natural crease in the eyelid. Save the darkest color to smudge a gentle line above the top lashes and below the bottom ones. To make eyes appear larger, the color should *not* meet at either the inner or outer corners of the eye.

5. As you smile, apply a touch of colored blush on the apples of your cheeks. Then use a bronzer to sweep color from these apples to your hairline. For a more sculpted facial look, apply bronzer to the forehead just beyond the tip of the eyebrows on your temples, and a light brushstroke down each side of your nose.

6. Apply mascara, line and color lips. (I am comfortable using commercial mascara because the product stays on lashes and is not applied to the skin where it could be absorbed.)

7. Set face with myrrh facial spritz.

DON'T FORGET YOUR NAILS

Nails are often the finishing touch of a beauty routine, but I rarely have time for a manicure. Instead, I try to keep my nails healthy and the cuticles moisturized. There are some natural ways to do this.

We learned from our chapter on hair that biotin, a B vitamin, is essential for producing keratin, the building block of gorgeous hair *and* nails. One study of biotin's effects on nails produced dramatic results: A Swiss study revealed that "taking a 2,500 mcg biotin supplement daily produced a 25 percent increase in nail thickness, leading 91 percent of the participants to say that after six months of use their nails looked better than ever."[2]

The study used supplements. Again, I prefer to add whole foods into my diet rather than try to remember to take a pill every day. Anytime you can add whole foods into your diet, your whole body will benefit. If your nails are weak and ragged, try adding these foods into your diet, which are among the top sources of biotin:

Nuts (almonds, walnuts)
Beans
Brewer's yeast

All of these foods were, of course, staples in the biblical age as well as our own. If you noticed brewer's yeast, and wondered why a beer-making by-product is on our list, you should realize that drinking beer was popular in biblical times. One ancient painting shows a couple drinking a large vat of beer together, through very long straws. It looks like an ancient version of two lovers sharing a soda. When King Solomon said "there's nothing new under the sun," he was right!

Also, for healthy nails and cuticles, be sure to keep moisturizer near your sinks, next to the hand soap, and moisturize your hands after washing.

THE TRUTH ABOUT "GETTING YOUR BEAUTY REST"

Sleep is a divine way to relieve stress and refresh our bodies, souls, and spirits. A good night's sleep rejuvenates us and boosts our immune system, our stress response, and even helps with weight control. Our bodies actively repair themselves at night; bodybuilders are known for needing extra sleep so their bodies can repair and build muscle. Our skin, too, is repairing itself and rejuvenating itself while we sleep. It's always a good idea to remove all makeup and nourish the skin before you get your beauty rest. In place of more expensive commercial products, here are a few suggestions you can try that will help create a soothing ritual that relaxes you, sending a message to your body that it is time for deep sleep.

BEDTIME ROUTINE

1. Thoroughly remove all makeup. I use olive oil to remove my eye makeup. It's nourishing to the skin and many commercial eye makeup removers have "soapy," drying ingredients, or petroleum-based formulations.

2. Use olive oil (or coconut oil), mixed with a dab of concealer under your eyes if dark circles are a problem. If you feel a bit pampered, and look a bit better, I think you'll be in a better mood for sweet sleep.

3. Be sure to moisturize the oft-neglected areas: hands, feet,

elbows, neck. (Keep nighttime moisturizers on your bedside table so you won't have to get out of bed if you realize you've forgotten to apply them.) I use coconut oil at night because it is such a rich skin moisturizer and has such a delicate fragrance.

4. Spritz yourself with a gently scented water, such as rosewater or lavender water. A little spritz with a soft scent relaxes you immediately and prepares you for rest.

5. Keep an ultrasonic humidifier by your bed. (We'll discuss this more in the next chapter.) Adding moisture to the bedroom air keeps your skin moisturized and also helps your breathing for a more restful sleep.

6. Keep a small book of nighttime devotions or uplifting meditations near the bed and make it the last thing you read before going to sleep. God's Word is alive and active, unlike any other book ever written (Heb. 4:12). While your body is repairing itself and preparing for a new day, your spirit can be ministered to as God's Word resonates through your sleep. And this sleep is a blessing of God, who promises to give it to you, as His beloved (Ps. 127:2).

7

Beauty Secrets: Perfumes and Scent

Scent is one of the most powerful beauty secrets I'll share with you. Smells are processed in the same area of the brain that we process and store emotions and memories. That's why we have such an immediate response to certain smells, with the emotion and memory coming back to us faster than the rational recognition of the smell. Smell can instantly set the mood and set our expectations. It also can instantly set our perception of another person or place, even subconsciously.

SPIRIT AND SCENT

There has never before been so much scientific research to unlock the secrets of scent and understand how it affects our emotions and mood. But long ago, God gave His people directions on incorporating scent into their spiritual lives, and we can benefit from this wisdom if we learn how to apply it to our lives today.

SCENTS OF THE TEMPLE

God created perfume recipes to be used in worship that were so special, no one was allowed to copy them or they would be "cut off" from their people. (Talk about penalties for copyright infringement!) When you walked into the ancient temple, you were immediately transported by the scent of the perfume to another place, a holy space. Perfume set the mood for worship and intimacy. It opened our hearts.

Scent was used in two ways in the temple and tabernacle: as a holy anointing oil and as an incense.

THE ANOINTING OIL

Moreover the LORD spoke to Moses, saying: "Also take for yourself quality spices—five hundred shekels of liquid myrrh, half as much sweet-smelling cinnamon (two hundred and fifty shekels), two hundred and fifty shekels of sweet-smelling cane, five hundred shekels of cassia, according to the shekel of the sanctuary, and a hin of olive oil. And you shall make from these a holy anointing oil, an ointment compounded according to the art of the perfumer. It shall be a holy anointing oil. With it you shall anoint the tabernacle of meeting and the ark of the Testimony; the table and all its utensils, the lampstand and its utensils, and the altar of incense; the altar of burnt offering with all its utensils, and the laver and its base. You shall consecrate them, that they may be most holy; whatever touches them must be holy. And you shall anoint Aaron and his sons, and consecrate them, that they may minister to Me as priests." (Exod. 30:22–30)

The anointing oil was to be made from myrrh, cinnamon, cane, cassia, and olive oil. I imagine that the scent smelled very much like a scent we would associate with Christmas. The oil consecrated the objects, making them holy to the Lord. It's a beautiful example of the foreshadowing of the Holy Spirit and His fragrant anointing on believers. When you came near the tabernacle, it had a definite scent. It was unmistakable and unique, never to be found elsewhere. It was the scent of holiness, of the pursuit and revelation of God.

THE INCENSE

And the LORD said to Moses: "Take sweet spices, stacte and onycha and galbanum, and pure frankincense with these sweet spices; there shall be equal amounts of each. You shall make of these an incense, a compound according to the art of the perfumer, salted, pure, and holy. And you shall beat some of it very fine, and put some of it before the Testimony in the tabernacle of meeting where I will meet with you. It shall be most holy to you. But as for the incense which you shall make, you shall not make any for yourselves, according to its composition. It shall be to you holy for the LORD. Whoever makes any like it, to smell it, he shall be cut off from his people." (Exod. 30: 34–38)

Burning incense was a fragrant entreaty to God. *The Anchor Bible Dictionary* states that, "The purpose of the regular morning and evening incense offerings at this altar is to secure the presence of God and his attention to man's prayer. The incense smoke carries the prayer to God, who is hopefully appeased when he smells the fragrant odor of the delicious incense"[1]

There were several ingredients mentioned above that we're unfamiliar with: Stacte either came from resin from a tree called the storax, or it was a form of myrrh. Onycha was a special perfume scent made from sea mollusks. (Mollusks were also the source of the famous purple dye in biblical days.) Galbanum was made from the resin of a plant native to Queen Esther's land of Persia (now Iran). Galbanum is still available to us today, and you can buy essential oil of galbanum. The combined fragrance was most likely a musky, deep, spicy scent.

Scent is used as a metaphor throughout the Bible:

Your prayers are a beautiful scent rising to God, like "golden bowls full of incense" (Rev. 5:8 NIV). An angel appeared to announce the impending birth of John the Baptist as incense was burned by the priest Zechariah. When the time for burning incense began, the angel appeared and assured the priest that his wife's prayers had been heard. Incense was seen as carrying our prayers to God.

To God, we are the sweet fragrance of Christ (2 Cor. 2:15 NIV).

The knowledge of Christ is a pleasing fragrance (2 Cor. 2:14 NIV).

It was customary to anoint yourself with scented oils as part of grooming. Later, being "anointed" also came to mean being filled with the Holy Spirit (Luke 4:18 NIV).

MAKING QUIET TIMES SPECIAL

Many Christians have not been exposed to using scents as part of our worship rituals, although clearly this was part of our earliest spiritual heritage. I attended a class once where the instructor used scent to set the mood, to create a "space" separate from the world so that students could focus completely and let go of their cares. The impact was immediate and soothing. Of course, this is probably a part of the genius behind God's invention of special incense that could only be used in the temple and tabernacle. It helped the people recognize the sacred space. It set their mood and helped them set aside outside cares and focus on the Lord.

We can use scent in our daily meditation time to help us lessen the distractions of the outside world and concentrate more fully on the business of listening for God. It's not mysticism or magic. We've seen how powerful scent can be, and that God designed us to respond emotionally to scent. Using a special scent for our quiet times can help us set the mood for quiet contemplation, and shutter our minds against all the other images and nagging thoughts. It reinforces that this time is separate from the daily routine. I use the same scented candle on our Sabbath that I use during my quiet times.

Scents popular for quiet moments include sandalwood, rose, ylang ylang, and of course, frankincense and myrrh. Frankincense is even said to be a symbol of the divine name of God.[2]

All of these scents can be found alone or in special blends. It's not important to use a "biblical" scent, although I love thinking about King Solomon or Mary smelling these same fragrances so long ago. What's important is that you choose a scent you love and keep it separate from everything else you use.

When you burn a scented candle, it's wonderful to reflect on the mysterious nature of faith and love. The scent surrounds you, though you cannot see, feel, or touch it. Yet you know it's there. You cannot describe where the scent or smoke goes, but you understand as the wax burns low that it is indeed being carried above.

BEAUTY AND SCENT

Since we're created to respond to scent, we know that we can use scent to make ourselves, and our environment, attractive and pleasing. Let me share with you some secrets about natural versus synthetic scents, and ways to use God's gift of scent to your advantage.

NATURAL VERSUS SYNTHETIC

Someone once pointed out the irony of paying for "real lemon oil" in our furniture polish while we're content to drink lemonade made from artificial lemon flavorings. When it comes to our bodies, we're often too ready to settle for synthetics. But just as we can intuitively tell the difference between a real rose and a silk one, I think our bodies are capable at some level of detecting the difference between real and synthetic scents. Most research done on scent-behavior-emotional cues is done using synthetic scents, so we know that we do respond to synthetics. They "work" to elicit a response. What is currently being debated and studied is whether using natural scents offers any additional benefits therapeutically. Can a scent from a living plant do more to heal and restore the body and mind than a synthetic scent? What we currently know about synthetic scents is that they can provoke irritation, including headaches and allergies. I've discovered a few tips I'll share with you that will allow you to bring scent into every area of your life without fear of allergic responses and chemical effects.

Fragrance is the number one cause for contact allergies from cosmetics.[3]

Because manufacturers are not required to disclose what the fragrance is made of, you'll probably never know what caused the reaction. And remember, "fragrance free" beauty products often contain fragrances to create a neutral scent.

EVERYDAY SCENTS YOU'LL LOVE

Body spray. Create your own body spray by combining natural spring water with a few drops of your favorite essential oil. (This also makes a healthy alternative to chemical room deodorizers. My absolute favorite room spray is simply a few drops of peppermint essential oil mixed with spring water. Wonderful!)

Body moisturizer. You can mix essential oils into your coconut oil or almond oil. Be careful to choose a nonirritating essential oil, such as rose. Simply add 2–3 drops into a few tablespoons of oil and mix. (Essential oils should be labeled to tell you which are good for application directly on the skin.)

Being careful to rub the oil on your pulse points, you will have a subtle delicate scent that invites people to lean in.

Body powder. You can make your own healthy body powder by mixing cornstarch with a few drops of essential oil. Make an extra batch to give away as gifts.

SETTING A ROMANTIC MOOD WITH SCENT

Scent can be used to enhance our beauty, and it can be used to make our intimate time more beautiful. If you're having trouble getting in the mood for romance, scent can be a powerful ally. Remember that scent bypasses other systems and activates the portion of your brain responsible for emotion and memory.

You can use scent to help you transport yourself emotionally to the place where you're ready to be unveiled and intimate. It's so difficult for women to transcend their daily routine at once and return to that sacred, quiet place within that safeguards desire and passion. Everything in our society, as much as it touts sexuality, inhibits intimacy. We're bombarded all day long with messages that we're only "sexy" if we look a certain way, dress a certain way, or weigh a certain number. *Sexy* is a word that describes everything from cars to furniture to computer systems. Sex is simply a product, and we wonder why we can't just press the "on" button. Don't feel bad if you need a little help getting in the mood sometimes. You've spent all day in a culture that inhibits intimacy, and you need to shake off the messages of the world, and center yourself again in the divine creation of God. Use the following to set the mood.

   1. Body scrub. You may try starting with a shower, or bath, and visualize the unhealthy messages and layers of the world washing away. A body scrub softens the skin and the scent relaxes you. Here's a recipe that incorporates scent to make you feel beautiful, and receptive to letting go of the day's frustrations.

SCENTED BODY SCRUB

¼ cup granulated sugar or salt (the coarse grains exfoliate your skin)
¼ cup coconut or almond oil
2–4 drops of your favorite essential oil

---

   2. Perfuming your body. It may come as a surprise that dousing yourself with synthetic perfumes may inhibit intimacy and attraction rather than increase it. Our bodies have pheromones, natural scents that work to attract others to us. Pheromone experts suggest that "one of the first steps you can take to make yourself more appealing to others is to stop over-bathing, over-deodorizing, and over-dousing with commercial scents."[4] After your shower, anoint yourself with a delicate perfume, reserved only for romantic rendezvous. Apply the scent sparingly, but in more spots than you typically would with a perfume. (There are natural perfumes available—check the Resource Guide for places to buy them.)

You can also add a few drops of your favorite essential oils to body oils such as almond or coconut, and let them double as a massage oil. Experiment to find the scent that encourages you to breathe deeply and melt into a different frame of mind.

3. *Perfuming bed linens.* In biblical times, it was common to perfume the bed before lovemaking. Common scents included myrrh, aloes, and cinnamon (Prov. 7:17). (When a recent study reported that men were attracted to the scent of cinnamon, a clever manufacturer wasted no time creating a lipstick infused with the scent of cinnamon, advertised with the promise you'll "attract a man"! The idea behind the lipstick is that if he gets close enough to smell your lips, he'll be subconsciously attracted to you. Please allow me to save you some money: if he's close enough to smell your lipstick, he's already attracted.)

Perfuming the sheets—again, delicately—makes the experience of lovemaking more memorable. In Song of Solomon 1:16, the lover's bed is described as verdant, lush with greenery, the smell of the cedar beams of the bed creating a forest around them. This sure beats a typical bedside today, where you're more likely to find athlete's foot spray than sheet perfume. We don't make going to bed an experience, either for lovemaking or sleeping.

To create a perfume for your sheets, simply mix a few drops of essential oil into spring water, and keep in a spritzer. (You can also make different varieties with scents that invoke feelings of relaxation and use them in guest bedrooms and linen closets.)

For romance, you may want to try deeper, richer scents. My favorite romantic scent, anise, has a rich, deep licorice smell, similar to the type linked to an increase in women's romantic desire.[5] I usually buy anise extract for this spray, which is available at any grocery store. Anise was popular with the ancient Babylonians and Egyptians, who prized it for its many applications.

ROMANTIC ANISE LINEN SPRAY

1 cup spring water
1 teaspoon anise extract (baking extract)

Pour into a small spritzer and shake. Keep in the refrigerator in between uses.

Remember, if anise is not a scent that appeals to you, simply experiment with different essential oil blends to find one that appeals to you. King Solomon's bed smelled like a verdant, lush forest, so you can try any number of plant-based scents.

4. Perfuming the air. A new way to perfume the bedroom, while also caring for your skin, is an ultrasonic humidifier. Essential oils can be added to the water, which is then dispersed by a fine vapor created by ultrasonic energy. I found a very reasonably priced version at Wal-Mart. These humidifiers work wonders in the winter, when heating systems dry out the air and parch our skin.

For more ways to incorporate scent into the bedroom, and throughout the home, consider adding candles and fresh fruits. Naturally scented candles are available and fragrance the environment without chemicals (see the Resource Guide). A bowl of fresh fruits is a beautiful addition to any décor. (You can also choose your candles to complement the scent of the fruits.)

Beauty, and scent, is about how we feel. Our inner state communicates to others and transforms our appearance into one of radiance. Scent is one more avenue by which we can tap into our secret selves, the beautiful lives that we want to share with the world.

Appendix A:
Host a Beauty Secrets
of the Bible *Party*

W ant a fun night of ministering to your friends, with no
unpleasant pressure to buy or sell products? You can share
the message and ministry of *Beauty Secrets of the Bible* with a
Beauty Secrets of the Bible Party!

There's nothing to sell and no pressure to buy—not even my
books. I am going to help you *give* everything away. You are going
to give away samples of the products we talk about in *Beauty
Secrets of the Bible* and share what you've learned about toxic commercial products. Together, we can educate women and transform
an industry that has made billions of dollars off of deception and
oppressive marketing tactics.

Beauty belongs first, and forever, to God. Here's your chance
to share this message with your friends and truly minister to
them. Let's tell them the truth about what's out there, because no
one else may. Let's give them incredible alternatives that they can
use for the rest of their lives. You won't sell anything—not even
this book. I'll give you all the information you need, for free.

Go online to my website at www.gingergarrett.com, and you

can download a free party kit. It contains invitations and information cards for many of the items and recipes listed in the book. You simply print your kit and purchase the products at your local grocery store that you'd like to sample that night. Olive oil as a moisturizer? I've got an information card packed with interesting highlights and health information. Want a snack to set out? Try the BSB Trail Mix, and pass out the recipe to your friends—I've included it in the party kit. Create a batch of the Rich Milk Cleanser and let women try it on their hands. Pass out the Ingredients to Watch For Checklist, and let women have a resource to help them read labels on their own products from home.

I promise it will be a fun night of trying products, laughing, and loving your friends. Best of all, you won't be selling anything. Just go have fun, and enjoy being one of the first women to start a revolution in the beauty care industry.

Appendix B: Resource Guide

RETAILERS

WAL-MART

Wal-Mart carries a huge variety of products that support the Beauty Secrets lifestyle at very reasonable prices.

Wal-Mart Shopping List

- ❖ Cosmetic bottles (located near the travel and trial sizes of grooming products)
- ❖ Ultrasonic humidifier (check near the pharmacy)
- ❖ Whole almonds (almonds out of the shell but with the brown skin on)
- ❖ Dried dates, figs, and raisins
- ❖ Olive oil
- ❖ Grapeseed oil
- ❖ Vinegar (pick up several varieties to experiment with for taste)
- ❖ Organic green tea
- ❖ Supplements: cinnamon and enteric-coated fish oil
- ❖ Makeup brushes for natural mineral makeup

❖ Aloe vera plant (buy two—one for kitchen and one for bath)
❖ Coffee grinder to use with fresh flaxseeds

WHOLE FOODS MARKET®

If you're planning a trip to your local market, stock up on these items:

❖ Essential oils
❖ Naturally scented candles
❖ Meyenberg powdered goat's milk
❖ Coconut, almond, and olive oil
❖ Pure fruit juices for extra antioxidants
❖ Vinegars
❖ In-season produce (pomegranates in fall and winter; figs in summer)
❖ Mineral makeups and other natural beauty products

PACKAGING

These sites offer a wonderful selection and great discounts for beautifully packaging your homemade products:

Specialty Bottle
www.specialtybottle.com

Spoil yourself with gorgeous containers for all your cosmetics, at incredible prices. Buy extras to give to friends.

Uline
www.uline.com

I buy plastic bags from Uline that can be used for scented bath salts or food gifts (such as the Beauty Secrets Trail Mix).

Wholesale Materials Suppliers

There is a huge market for women who want to create their own natural cosmetics for personal and commercial use. These are two companies I've dealt with that are exceptional finds:

The Chemistry Store
www.chemistrystore.com

A supplier of Dead Sea salts, containers, and fun additives such as glitters to make fabulous gift sets. The prices are truly reasonable and this would make a great project for a ministry, Christmas gifts, or a home-based business.

Somerset Cosmetics Company
www.makingcosmetics.com

This company has been in business for years and is geared toward supplying wholesale materials for those wishing to create their own line of cosmetics. If you've ever thought about starting your own line of beauty care products, this company can supply elegant, professional materials that will make your finished products stand out. You can even sign up for a free newsletter with "recipes" and tips.

Cosmetics Resources

General Information and Safety Concerns

Campaign for Safe Cosmetics
www.safecosmetics.org

The Environmental Working Group
www.ewg.org

Provides an easy-to-use database of commercial products and potential toxins. You can search by product name or category, and also sign up for a monthly newsletter.

MINERAL POWDERS AND NATURAL COSMETICS

Emani
www.Emani.com

Michelle Doan, founder and artistic director, has an intuitive eye for color and her loose minerals are wonderful—free of preservatives, artificial fragrances, and irritating, pore-blocking ingredients.

Bare Escentuals
www.bareminerals.com

You've probably seen this line advertised on television or sold in stores. You can usually find a store near you to try the products before you buy. You can shop online or get information on finding a retailer near you on the website.

Jane Iredale
www.janeiredale.com

Jane Iredale mineral cosmetics are sold through spas and medical offices. For a location near you, or for more extensive information on mineral cosmetics, visit the website. I love her pressed mineral powder—it's one of the few that does not contain talc. It's great for women who are trying minerals for the first time.

Burt's Bees
www.burtsbees.com

Burt's Bees, a pioneer in natural body care, is launching a line of natural lipsticks and glosses. They are the best I've ever tried—never drying, long lasting, and beautifully tinted. You can find Burt's Bees almost anywhere these days, from Whole Foods Market® to gift shops.

NUTRITIONAL SUPPORT

Dr. Don Colbert
www.drcolbert.com

Dr. Colbert helped pioneer the idea that the diet Jesus ate, now often referred to as a "Mediterranean" diet, is also the most effective strategy for creating good health and vitality. The author of dozens of books, including the bestseller *What Would Jesus Eat?* with an accompanying cookbook, you can find more information about his work and ministry at his website.

Dr. Carrie Carter
www.carteronhealth.com

Carrie Carter, M.D., F.A.A.P, has been a board-certified primary care physician for over sixteen years. Dr. Carter provides medically sound information about women's health issues, including disease prevention, nutrition, and menopause. Her engaging and understandable woman-to-woman style makes her a practical resource you'll turn to frequently—just as you'd turn to a trusted friend for help.

Pure Fruit Technologies
www.purefruittechnologies.com

Dr. Wayne Geilman is the technical director for this company, which specializes in exotic juices that pack a powerful punch of antioxidants. I use their Goji-Zen and Mango-Xan juices to make sure I get plenty of antioxidants each day.

Spectrum Organics
www.spectrumorganics.com

Spectrum offers a wide variety of cooking oils, salad dressings, and nutritional supplements. I use their organic coconut oil for body and hair care, and recommend their organic olive oil and apple cider vinegar as well. Spectrum is usually available in the health foods section of your local grocery store.

Dr. Andrew Weil
www.drweil.com

Dr. Weil is a respected doctor who has created a wealth of resources for those seeking more natural solutions to healthy living. You can find more information about his work, including Weil Supplements, on his website. I use his brand of supplements, which includes evening primrose and fish oils, and feel very confident that the supplements are manufactured correctly and offer a good value.

SKIN AND BODY CARE

Kimberly Sayer
www.kimberlysayer.com

Kimberly Sayer is an organic chemist with an advanced expertise in selecting her harvest for her products. They are preserved with a natural preservative system, not parabens. I am in love with her cleanser and lavender toner. They smell divine.

Christopher Watt
www.christopherwatt.com

Spa expert and facialist to the stars, Christopher also offers his expertise to everyone—check out his website for great ideas and recipes. If you're ever in West Hollywood, treat yourself to a visit at his luxurious spa.

Jackson-Mitchell's Meyenberg Goat Milk Products
www.meyenberg.com

I buy my powdered goat's milk from Meyenberg Milk and love it. It's inexpensive when you consider that a can will last for about six to eight weeks when part of a beauty regimen. I find it at my local Whole Foods Market®, but you can also ask your grocery store manager to order it, or buy it online.

Max Green Alchemy
www.maxgreenalchemy.com

Max Green offers a number of natural products for hair and body care. Their shampoo and conditioner are so refreshing; I swish my hair throughout the day just to breathe in the sweet aroma of rosemary and herbs.

Motherlove Herbal Company
www.motherlove.com

Founded by Kathryn Higgins, this company is primarily for nursing and new moms. I was shocked to discover that my baby's diaper cream contained parabens. Motherlove produces a wonderful, paraben-free diaper cream.

Aubrey Organics
www.aubrey-organics.com

Aubrey is a market leader in organic skin and body care. Aubrey also has a line of natural perfumes.

Zia Natural Skincare
www.zianatural.com

Zia is responding proactively to the paraben issue and introducing more products that are paraben-free. I love two products in particular: The Ultimate "C" Serum and the Deep Moisture Repair Serum.

SeaOra Mineral Skin Care
www.SeaOra.com

SeaOra® offers products from the Dead Sea. It's hard to find a company that sells 100% Dead Sea Mud, and SeaOra does. I love the fact that they list ingredients for every product, so that consumers can make an informed choice.

ESSENTIAL OILS AND CANDLES

Aroma Rx
www.Aromarx.com

Michele Williams, RPh, founder and president, offers hundreds of oils and blends. She also is the author of *Only the*

Essentials, a no-nonsense guide to understanding and employing aromatherapy in your life.

Aura Cacia
www.auracacia.com

Aura Cacia is available at most Whole Foods Markets® and provides essential oils and body oils such as almond oil, apricot kernel oil, and sesame oil.

Aroma Naturals Candles
www.aromanaturals.com

This candle company uses essential oils in their lovely candles and uses frankincense, blended with lavender or patchouli, in two popular scents. I've found these candles to be long lasting and to have wonderful, fresh fragrances.

STRENGTH TRAINING

These sites give you great information from trusted sources:

www.joycevedral.com
www.drpeeke.com
www.bodyforlife.com

CHARITABLE GIVING—HUNGER RELIEF

Check www.charitywatch.org for ratings of charities to find out how much of your money actually goes to feeding the needy. All of these charities had high ratings as of June 2006:

Bread for the World
www.bread.org

Action Against Hunger
www.actionagainsthunger.org

Food for Survival
www.foodforsurvival.org

Freedom From Hunger
www.freefromhunger.org/about

The Hunger Project
www.thp.org

CHARITABLE GIVING—HUNGER RELIEF AND CHRISTIAN MINISTRY

Samaritan's Purse
www.samaritanspurse.org

Samaritan's Purse is a charitable organization with an emphasis on programs that provide food and emergency relief to children around the world. Request their Gifts of Hope catalog for your Christmas shopping!

Feed The Hungry
www.feedthehungry.org

Feed the Hungry distributes food all over the world, using local networks of churches and pastors so that those in need are fed physically and spiritually.

Acknowledgments

This book started out as a magazine article. It was Lee Hough of Alive Communications who asked me to consider creating it as a book. Lee, as usual, your advice was spot-on. You're a good man to show enthusiasm for my thoughts on facials and wrinkle creams. It's been my goal to write a book worthy of the job you did representing me.

This book was also greatly enriched by the experts who graciously gave of their time and expertise. I owe each of them a debt of gratitude.

I am also indebted to Thomas Nelson Publishers, especially Brian Hampton, who took a chance on the project and patiently listened to me talking about beauty products he had never tried, and never would. Every person at Thomas Nelson has been a blessing to this project and I am truly thankful for the opportunity to work with you all, including Paula Major, Kristen Parrish, Belinda Bass, Kristen Vasgaard, Brandi Lewis, Jennifer Greenstein, and Pamela Clements. Thanks also to the creative team, including Kirk DouPonce and photographer Don Sparks.

And an additional thank-you to the SMU Women's Studies Department.

And of course, a big thanks to my family and friends who have supported this project with their time, kind words, prayers, and enthusiasm: My sister-in-law Andi experimented endlessly with the products I created for her and was selfless in her support. My dear friend Carolynn James helped me perfect my original presentation and was a constant encouragement. My mom and grandmom prayed for me and cheered me on.

Lastly, I want to thank those who make writing possible for me. My team includes my incredible husband Mitch, and my parents, who all pitch in when I need to travel or do interviews. I also have a group of advisors that surround me with wisdom and encouragement: the Reinoehls, the Jameses, Sherrill McCracken, the Linnabarys, the Crazes, the Dosses, and the Sittons. I thank you so much for your prayers. And, for the girls of NPCC who are my beloved friends: Gidget Johnson, Tina Wheeler, DeDe Davis, Kelly Arrington, Susan Dotson, Ginny Haynie, Karetha Milton, Amy Davis, Andrea Jones, and Kathy Harold.

Notes

CHAPTER I
1. "Vital Stats." *Health,* April 2005, 180.

CHAPTER 2
1. Michael Capuzzo, *Close to Shore* (New York: Broadway Books, 2001), 48.
2. Joan Jacobs Brumberg, *The Body Project: An Intimate History of American Girls* (New York: Vintage Books, 1998), xx.
3. *The St. James Encyclopedia of Pop Culture* (Gale Group, 2002), s.v. "Flappers."
4. Brumberg, xxv.
5. Debra Waterhouse, M.P.H., R.D., *Outsmarting The Female Fat Cell* (New York: Hyperion, 1993), 2.
6. Geneen Roth, *Appetites: On the Search for True Nourishment* (New York: Plume, 1997), 14.
7. Shannon Brownlee, "Are These Diet Pills Deadly?" *Glamour,* February 1, 2003, http://www.newamerica.net/publications/articles/2003/are_these_diet_pills_deadly (accessed on December 1, 2006).
8. Russ Mason, M.S., "Exploring the Potentials of Human Olfaction: An Interview with Alan R. Hirsch, M.D., F.A.C.P.," *Alternative & Complementary Therapies,* Volume II, no. 3 (June 2005).
9. "The Super-Sizing of America," reported by John Nichols, Iowa Public Television, http://www.iptv.org/mtom/archivedfeature.cfm?Fid=215 (accessed May 27, 2006).

10. "Vital Stats." *Health*, December 2004, 176.

11. Food and Research Action Center, "Number of Hungry and Food Insecure Americans Jumps to 38 Million in 2004," news release, Friday, October 28, 2005, http://www.frac.org/Press_Release/10.28.05.html.

12. "Hunger Facts," Bread for the World & Bread for the World Institute, http://www.bread.org/learn/hunger-basics/ (accessed May 27, 2006).

13. Ibid.

14. Marianne McGinnis, "Weight Loss News: Snack on This." *Prevention*, February 2003, 77.

15. Anne Underwood and Jerry Adler, "What You Don't Know About Fat." *Newsweek*, August 23, 2004, 42.

16. Kelly Brownell, "Yo-yo dieting: repeated efforts to lose weight can give you a hefty problem," *Psychology Today*, January 1988, http://www.findarticles.com/p/articles/mi_m1175/is_n1_v22/ai_6213713 (accessed October 16, 2006).

17. David Noel Freedman, ed., *The Anchor Bible Dictionary.* (New York: Random House, 1992).

18. Ibid.

19. The Almond Board of California, "Almonds Are In!" The Almond Board of California, http://www.almondsarein.com/Health Professionals/content.cfm?ItemNumber=1626 (accessed December 1, 2006).

20. The World's Healthiest Foods, "Almonds," The George Mateljan Foundation, http://www.whfoods.org/genpage.php?tname=food spice&dbid=20#descr (accessed May 24, 2006).

21. Ibid.

22. Ibid.

23. Ibid.

24. "Foods That Soothe Swollen Cells." *First*, January 30, 2006, 27.

25. Amy Scholten, MPH, McLean Hospital, "Omega-3 Fatty Acids and Mental Health," http://healthlibrary.epnet.com/getcontent .aspx?token=d291a9f5-2226-447d-88bf-2cb7e6905ec3&docid=/ healthy/mind/2003/omegamental (accessed October 16, 2006).

26. "Cinnamon, Cloves Improve Insulin Function, Lower Risk Factors for Diabetes, Cardiovascular Disease," Medical News Today, http://www.medicalnewstoday.com/medicalnews.php?newsid=41026# (accessed May 27, 2006).

27. Ibid.

28. Ibid.

29. Ibid.

30. Freedman.

31. The World's Healthiest Foods, "Figs," The George Mateljan Foundation, http://www.whfoods.com/genpage.php?tname=food spice&dbid=24 (accessed May 27, 2006).

32. Janet Raloff, "Vinegar As A Sweet Solution?" *Science News Online*, http://www.sciencenews.org/articles/20041218/food.asp (accessed June 8, 2006).

33. "Foods That Soothe Swollen Cells." *First*, January 30, 2006, 27.

CHAPTER THREE

1. Judith E. Foulke, "Cosmetic Ingredients: Understanding the Puffery," *FDA Consumer*, http://www.fda.gov/fdac/reprints/puffery.html (accessed July 15, 2006).

2. Ibid.

3. Ibid.

4. Environmental Working Group, "Skin Deep," Environmental Working Group October 2005 Report, http://www.ewg.org/issues/siteindex/issues.php?issueid=5005. (This article can only be accessed by subscribers.)

5. "Are Your Products Safe?" The Campaign for Safe Cosmetics, http://www.safecosmetics.org/your_health.

6. Marianne Marchese, "Environmental influences on women's health: how to avoid endocrine disrupting compounds," *Townsend Letter for Doctors and Patients*, July 2004, http://www.findarticles.com/p/articles/mi_m0ISW/is_252/ai_n6112832 (accessed March 21, 2006).

7. P. D. Darbre, A. Aljarrah, W. R. Miller, N. G. Coldham, M. J. Sauer, and G. S. Pope, "Concentrations of Parabens in Human Breast Tumours," *Journal of Applied Toxicology* 24, no. 1 (January 2004).

8. Steve Connor, "Men being emasculated by toiletries," *The (London) Independent*, October 7, 1998, http://www.findarticles.com/p/articles/mi_qn4158/is_19981007/ai_n14195897.

9. "Diethanolamine and Cosmetic Products," U.S. Food and Drug Administration, December 1999, revised 2006, http://www.cfsan.fda.gov/~dms/cos-dea.html (accessed January 11, 2007).

10. "Preliminary Study of Phthalate Exposure in Humans Finds Association with Sperm DNA Damage," Harvard School of Public Health, December 10, 2002, www.hsph.harvard.edu/press/releases/press12102202.html (accessed January 11, 2007).

11. Russ Hauser, Harvard School of Public Health, http://www.hsph.harvard.edu/faculty/RussHauser.html (accessed January 11, 2007).

12. "Phthalates and Cosmetic Products," U.S. Food and Drug Administration, http://www.cfscan.fda.gov/~dms/cos-phth.html (accessed July 15, 2006).

13. "Drugs & Supplements: Horse Chestnut (Aesculus hippocastanum L.)," Mayo Clinic.com, http://www.mayoclinic.com/health/horse-chestnut/NS_patient-Horsechestnut #E5944815-E7FF-0DBD-1A526394DBB71D91 (accessed October 14, 2006).

14. "Ingredients for Ethnic Skin and Hair," *Homemade Cosmetics Update*, no. 12, June 2005, http://www.makingcosmetics.com/newsletters/n12-newsletter-june-05.pdf.

15. *Columbia Encyclopedia*, s.v. "Petroleum Maturation."

16. "Recordkeeping Requirements for Human Food and Cosmetics Manufactured From, Processed With, or Otherwise Containing, Material From Cattle," U.S. Department of Health and Human Services, Food and Drug Administration, July 14, 2004, http://www.fda.gov/OHRMS/DOCKETS/98fr/04-15880.htm (accessed July 15, 2006).

17. Carol Lewis, "Clearing Up Cosmetic Confusion," *FDA Consumer*, May–June 1998, revised August 2000, http://www.fda.gov/fdac/features/1998/398_cosm.html (accessed July 15, 2006).

18. Ibid.

CHAPTER FOUR

1. J.W. White, Jr. and Landis W. Doner, Honey Composition and Properties, *"Beekeeping in the United States," Agriculture Handbook*, no. 335, revised October 1980, http://www.beesource.com/pov/usda/beekpUSA82.htm (accessed April 24, 2006).

2. American Academy of Dermatology, "Vitamins To Protect Against And Reverse Aging: The Truth vs. The Tall Tales," American Academy of Dermatology, February 25, 2002, http://www.aad.org/public/News/NewsReleases/Press+Release+Archives/Cosmetic+Dermatology +-+Aging/TopicalVitamins.htm (accessed October 7, 2006).

3. Nicholas Perricone, M.D., *The Perricone Promise* (New York: Time Warner, 2004). 44.

4. Ibid.

5. Dr. Andrew Weil, "Are Nuts a Healthy Nibble?" May 31, 2004, http://www.drweil.com/drw/u/id/QAA326631 (accessed October 16, 2006).

6. Emily Crawford, "The Ancient Pomegranate Promises A New Path to

Good Health," *Columbia News Service,* May 3, 2004, http://www.jrn.columbia.edu/studentwork/cns/2004-05-03/763.asp (accessed June 24, 2006).

7. Indo-Asian News Service, "Eat more fruits, vegetables to avoid wrinkles," *RxPG News,* April 18, 2006, http://www.rxpgnews.com/ health/food/article_4065.shtml (accessed October 7, 2006).

8. Barry Callebaut, "The History of Chocolate, 1500–today," Brown's Hand Made Chocolates, http://www.brownes.co.uk/acatalog/ History.html (accessed July 17, 2006).

9. Sally Wadyka, "Change Your Beauty Destiny," *Shape,* February 2005, http://www.findarticles.com/p/articles/mi_m0846/is_6_24/ai_n948201 4 (accessed October 7, 2006).

10. Sharon Bahrych, "Your Prayer Life Does Make a Difference," *Vibrant Life,* November 2000, http://www.findarticles.com/p/articles/ mi_m0826/is_6_16/ai_67325748 (accessed October 16, 2006).

11. "Higher exercise intensity, lower stress - GetFit News," *Shape,* December 2003, http://www.findarticles.com/p/articles/mi_m0846/ is_4_23/ai_111146660 (accessed October 16, 2006).

12. Miranda Hitti, "Obesity, Smoking Linked to Faster Aging," *WebMD,* June 15, 2005, http://onhealth.webmd.com/script/main/art.asp? articlekey=56189.

13. Kimberly Beauchamp, ND, "Honey Mixture Improves Skin Conditions," Bastyr Center for Natural Health, http://www. bastyrcenter.org/content/view/422 (accessed October 19, 2006).

14. Anne Harding, "Olive Oil Ingredient May Improve Circulation," Yahoo News, November 28, 2005, http://naooa.mytradeassociation.org/ hottopics/olive-oil-may-protect-aga.shtml (accessed March 21, 2006).

15. Sarah Mahoney, "The Real-Life Stress Survival Guide," *Prevention,* http://www.prevention.com/article/0,5778,s1-1-65-209-6113 -1-P,00.html (accessed July 15, 2006).

16. David Noel Freedman, ed., *The Anchor Bible Dictionary.* (New York: Random House, 1992).

17. Jon Fogg, "Frankincense Shows Promise in Fighting Skin Cancer," Fox News, February 3, 2006, http://www.foxnews.com/story/ 0,2933,183778,00.html (accessed October 10, 2006).

CHAPTER FIVE

1. Audrey T. Hingley, "OTC Options: Controlling Dandruff," *FDA Consumer,* http://www.fda.gov/bbs/topics/CONSUMER/ CON0290d.html (accessed March 21, 2006).

2. Theresa Anne Morin, "1-ingredient beauty fixes: these simple, inexpensive remedies soften dry skin, control dandruff, and more in no time–Do-It-Yourself Cures," *Natural Health*, September 2003, http://www.findarticles.com/p/articles/mi_m0NAH/is_7_33/ai_107637 378/print (accessed March 21, 2006).

3. Hingley.

4. S.M. Innis and D.B. Allardyce, "Possible biotin deficiency in adults receiving long-term total parenteral nutrition," *American Journal of Clinical Nutrition* 37, February 1983: 185-187.

5. Karyn Siegel-Maier, "Natural, nutritional nail care," *Better Nutrition*, April 1999, http://www.findarticles.com/p/articles/mi_m0FKA/ is_4_61/ai_54245772.

6. "Flaxseed Slows Down Hair Loss." *Woman's World*, November 1, 2005, 13.

7. A.S. Rele, R.B. Mohile, "Effect of mineral oil, sunflower oil, and coconut oil on prevention of hair damage," *Journal of Cosmetic Science* 54, no. 2 (March–April 2003): 175-92.

CHAPTER SIX

1. Wendell L. Combest, Ph.D., "Aloe Vera, " *U.S. Pharmacist*, http://www.uspharmacist.com/oldformat.asp?url=newlook/files/Alte/apr 00aloe.cfm&pub_id=8&article_id=503 (accessed June 24, 2006).

2. "The 'Inner' Secret to Strong, Lovely Hair." *First for Women*, March 13, 2006, 12.

CHAPTER SEVEN

1. David Noel Freedman, ed., *The Anchor Bible Dictionary*. (New York: Random House, 1992).

2. Suzetta Tucker, "ChristStory Christmas Symbols: Frankincense." *ChristStory Christian Bestiary*, 1999, http://ww2.netnico.net/users/ legend01/frankin.htm (accessed March 4, 2006).

3. "Allergies to Cosmetics Ingredients," *Homemade Cosmetics Update*, no. 9, March 2005, http://www.makingcosmetics.com/newsletters/ n09-newsletter-march-05.pdf.

4. Stacy Short, "The Scent of Seduction: How to Use Scent to Your Advantage in the Game of Love," The Smell & Taste Treatment and Research Foundation, http://www.scienceofsmell.com/ scienceofsmell/index.cfm?action=scentsofseduction (accessed October 16, 2006).

5. Alan R. Hirsch, M.D., *ScentSational Sex: The Secret to Using Aroma For Arousal* (Boston, MA: Element Books, 1998), 102.

About the Author

Ginger Garrett is the author of the critically acclaimed *Chosen: The Lost Diaries of Queen Esther* (nominated for the 2006 Christian Book Award) and *Dark Hour*. An expert in ancient women's lives, she loves to create relevant resources that help modern women understand their forgotten sisters. You can visit her website at www.gingergarrett.com.

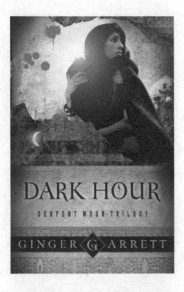

Dark Hour
by Ginger Garrett
1-57683-869-2

An expertly woven tapestry of stunning betrayal, bloodthirsty revenge, and fiery passion sets the stage for an epic of mothers and daughters, sisters and brothers, husbands and wives.

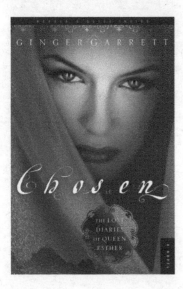

Chosen
by Ginger Garrett
1-57683-651-7

She came to conquer a king but discovered a man and, in the end, saved a nation. What really happened in Xerxes' palace? Queen Esther's secret diaries tell all.

To order copies, visit your local Christian bookstore, call NavPress at 1-800-366-7788, or log on to www.navpress.com.

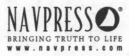

NAVPRESS
BRINGING TRUTH TO LIFE
www.navpress.com

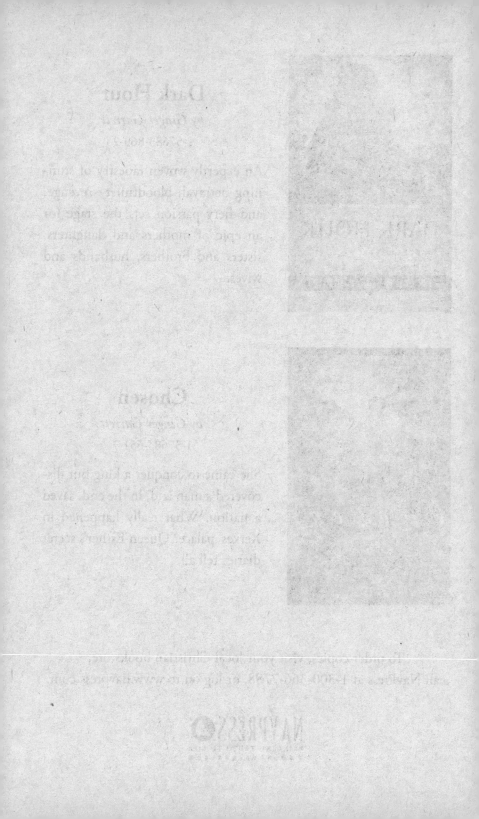